MANAGEMENT SIMULATIONS

For Mental Health & Human Services Administration

MICHAEL J. AUSTIN

THE HAWORTH PRESS

NEW YORK

The Haworth Press, 149 Fifth Avenue, New York, New York 10010

Library of Congress Cataloging in Publication Data

Austin, Michael J
   Management simulations for mental health and
human services administration.

   Includes bibliographies.
   1. Mental health services--Administration.
2. Mental health services--Administration--Problems,
exercises, etc. I. Title. [DNLM: 1. Community
mental health services--Organization and administration. 2. Social work--Organization and administration. WM30.3 A937m]
RA790.5.A95   658'.91'3622   78-12172
ISBN 0-917724-07-0

Printed in the United States of America

TABLE OF CONTENTS

PREFACE

    The commitment to prepare and upgrade mental health and human service administrators for leadership and managerial competence serves as the inspiration for developing this series of management simulations. Such a commitment developed over the past decade in which practitioners and students alike commented on the continuous "lack of fit" between theory and practice. This observation grew into a plea for help: "Can't you give us something that will allow us to practice what you preach?" These simulations therefore represent an effort to begin to bridge the gap between theory and practice.

    Useful as part of a management skills laboratory or a continuing education workshop, these simulations emphasize both content and process. The content of each simulation reflects a series of theoretical concepts along with basic information about agency or program operations. The basic premise for the emphasis on content is Lewin's famous comment, "There's nothing more practical than a good theory."

    The emphasis on process in each simulation results from a strong desire to incorporate skill development as a major focus for all simulations. While there has been considerable interest and activity in developing games for training purposes, it was felt that simulations as structured exercises would provide more attention to skill development than the "win-lose" orientation of games. The structure of each simulation includes time limits for each activity. While these limits may be somewhat arbitrary, they reflect the constant time pressures which plague busy administrators.

Another premise which underlies the development of these simulations is the idea that some people "learn best by doing." The actual completion of a simulated activity provides the immediate feedback not often found in either classroom or agency experience. People who choose to work in the fields of mental health and human services often bring with them considerable interpersonal skills. This series of simulations is designed to build upon those skills.

The topics selected for each simulation were based upon several criteria. First, each simulation represents a situation which rarely surfaces during the internship or field experience of a student preparing for mental health and human service administration. Similarly, they represent situations which experienced direct service practitioners, promoted into administrative positions, have rarely experienced. Secondly, the themes of each simulation are rarely found in texts on mental health and human service administration in a form by which the learner can test his or her knowledge and skills. There has been only limited success in the use of case materials in mental health and human service administration. This lack of success is based, in part, on the shortage of quality case studies and the ever-changing nature of program management.

One of the characteristics of our human condition is the general reluctance on the part of most people to take risks. We say that this is "human nature," but we also recognize that much of our behavior is learned from parents, friends, colleagues, or others. Therefore, it has become increasingly important to learn how to take risks. The structured learning activities of each simulation include situations which require risk-taking behavior. Like the airplane pilot in training who sits in a simulated cockpit to learn how to fly, current and future administrators can learn from specially designed simulations. It is impossible to crash but it is possible to take the risks necessary to learn how to handle difficult situations.

In a similar fashion, we have discovered that we can acquire insights into ourselves through the process of learning from others, especially our peers. Peer learning is a basic component of each simulation since participants must work together in order to do effective problem solving. These collaborative experiences also simulate the real life situations in agencies which rely heavily upon staff cooperation and coordination.

Since we are all students of administration, these simulations may be used by a wide variety of people, from the student preparing for a middle management position to an experienced practitioner desiring to refine his or her skills. While these simulations were designed to fit into a graduate curriculum in social administration, they can be useful in a wide variety of in-service training and continuing education workshop situations. It is assumed that each participant will read basic materials in human service administration in conjunction with the simulations (Anderson, Frieden, & Murphy, 1977; Slavin, 1978). For example, a basic knowledge of human service organizations would include familiarity with the following concepts: people processing organizations, agency environment, executive leadership, organizational goals and technology, authority and control, professionals and paraprofessionals, organization-client relations, interorganizational relations, evaluating organizational performance, and organizational innovation and change (Hasenfeld & English, 1974). Related to such knowledge components of administration are the skill components of planning, organizing, staffing, directing, coordinating, reporting, budgeting, and evaluating (Ehlers, Austin, & Prothero, 1976). In addition to basic knowledge and skills, it is important to acquire specialized knowledge of programs and agency structures throughout the human service field. For example, the knowledge and skill components of administration take on a special meaning in managing mental health services when it comes to planning, budgeting, personal management, financing, management information systems, intraorganizational and interorganizational relations, community participation, governmental systems, program innovations, and program evaluation (Feldman, 1973). Additional themes and readings are suggested in each simulation for those interested in learning more about specialized areas.

The simulations are organized into two types. The first six simulations emphasize management skills which can be applied in any area of human services. While the examples are primarily from mental health, the instructor and participants should be able to demonstrate applications to the fields of corrections, welfare, mental retardation, vocational rehabilitation, health care, and education. Four simulations are more in-depth approaches to four different organizational settings: a nonprofit county mental health association; a nonprofit voluntary community treatment facility (halfway house); a public multiprogram community agency (comprehensive community mental health center); and a large public total institution (state mental hospital). Parallels to these agencies are found in prisons, delinquency halfway houses, training schools for the retarded, sheltered workshops for the vocationally and physically disabled, and multiprogram public welfare departments. Each simulation can be described as follows:

1. Values and Ethics. Administrators may well experience conflict between their personal and professional goals and values. A goal of this simulation is to highlight the potential for such conflict and to emphasize the importance of recognizing it. Two assessment instruments enable participants to gain insights into their management values and philosophies. A third assessment instrument provides feedback and a model which enables the participant to become an effective member of a small task-oriented group.

2. Handling Conflict. Conflicts which arise within the work setting (both among staff as well as between clients and staff) demand the administrator's and supervisor's time and attention. This simulation structures experiences toward the resolution of defined conflict through planned action strategies.

3. Teaching Staff. This simulation is designed to teach trainees about staff development as related to the implementation of a therapeutic community. Major objectives include knowledge of training techniques and sequencing of learning tasks, knowledge of adult learning, knowledge of organizational change and the implementation of change, knowledge of resistance to change and how to deal with it, and knowledge of the therapeutic community concept as related to patient care.

4. Financial Analysis. This simulation is designed to facilitate the development of skills related to the following: (1) budget analysis (including projections of line-item and program budget); (2) development of fiscal alternatives (e.g., contingency budgets for both excess anticipated and reduced anticipated funds); (3) "costing out" of patient/client services and care; and (4) development of agency and program objectives versus budgetary goals.

5. Grievance. This simulation focuses on potential grievance issues which may be of concern to administrators in human service organizations. The simulation is designed to assist participants in defining sources of grievance, handling the process of formal grievance procedures, developing strategies for handling grievances, analyzing possible outcomes related to grievance procedures, and implementing strategies for resolving grievances.

6. Maxras. This simulation is designed as a child mental health service management simulation which directs participants to examine the forces which work upon social service agencies and influence their decision-making procedures. Participants, through their simulation experience, engage in case management and case coordination, plan referral processes, maintain client information systems, plan future budgets based on service information of prior years, and strategize in budget presentations in order to maximize agency survival.

7. Hanplan. This first of four substantive simulations is a planning simulation based on a voluntary mental health association. Participants engage in planning activities serving in the roles of executive director, lay board members, and the board chairman. Hanplan focuses on issues of executive-board relationships within a voluntary agency, goal setting within an organization, assessment of community needs, and the development of program priorities and service alternatives.

8. Halfway. This simulation places each participant in the position of the executive director or a key staff person in a psychiatric halfway house. It focuses on the need to integrate client and community objectives in order to provide effective client services while maintaining good community relations.

9. _Mancom_. This simulation provides participants with experiences relevant to the management of small and medium sized comprehensive community mental health centers. Learning experiences include understanding one's own personal style of management, gaining knowledge of an urban community mental health center, prioritizing key administrative tasks, deriving goals and objectives through the involvement of senior staff, demonstrating leadership skills in client and staff relations, and assessing one's own managerial self.

10. _Thronateeska_. This simulation provides participants with experiences in the management of large, state-operated mental health institutions. Through the simulation experiences, participants engage in selected administrative tasks including priority ranking of administrative issues, clarification of job responsibilities, development of effective community relations, and mediating peer conflict.

The ten simulations are based on the use of experiential exercises including role playing, in-basket techniques, and leaderless groups. The emphasis is on individual and group decision making in the context of real-life mental health and human service agency management situations. Simulation participants will learn the most from each simulation if they reflect a willingness: (1) to learn from peers; (2) to take risks; (3) to engage in each activity conscientiously; (4) to reflect a positive and flexible approach to learning; and (5) to avoid as much as possible the need for competition.

Accompanying the text is an _Instructor's Guide_ which identifies practical suggestions for the use of the simulations and a sample participant evaluation form. With particular emphasis on the instructor role, each simulation is then described in terms of learning objectives, possible modifications of the simulation format, suggestions regarding the debriefing section of each simulation, and references for further study.

The potential range of student and faculty interest in management simulations includes nursing, social work, psychology, psychiatry, guidance and counseling, vocational rehabilitation, corrections, special education, and health care administration. In social work alone, there are over 80 graduate programs with either a course or a sequence of courses related to middle-management training.

Similarly, departments of psychology offer graduate training in community psychology and psychiatry departments offer training in administrative psychiatry. In addition to the graduates, there are undergraduate students in health care administration, special education, and corrections who would benefit from the simulations. And finally, agency practitioners participating in workshops can gain new insights and skills from the completion of these simulations.

EVALUATING ADMINISTRATIVE COMPETENCE

Since the flood of human service legislation of the 1960s, there has been a renewed interest in the problems confronting the human service administrator. Despite this interest, most human service administrators who assume their first middle management position have rarely had the opportunity to acquire formal education in administration. On-the-job training has usually consisted of learning by doing supplemented occasionally by workshops, institutes, and continuing education courses.

Courses offered through continuing education or through formal degree programs often neglect the ongoing struggle to define competent administrative practice. What is a competent human service or mental health administrator? What values should such an administrator possess? What tasks do administrators perform? Answers to these questions involve the ability to assess the knowledge, skills, and values as related to administrative performance. While existing measurement instruments often prove to be inadequate, there is increasing interest in measuring administrative behavior through situational tests. Some industries, state governments, and local school systems are turning to measuring responses to certain situations as a way of assessing new candidates for management potential. The assessment procedure simulates "live" managerial situations and attempts to develop information about potential for performance at a variety of administrative levels. It combines several predictors of managerial success including written psychological tests (alone these have proven ineffective), extensive individual interviews, and a series of situational tests. The situational tests have been found to correlate highly with successful performance.

In developing the situations for assessment, considerable emphasis is placed on defining the performance criteria most closely related to the job for which a candidate is being considered. The situational test is then designed based upon these performance criteria. The following types of situational tests provided some of the basic ideas reflected in this training text:

1. Management games that simulate an organization and are designed to require the use of basic principles of management. The players are observed by an assessor who rates them on their behavior.

2. The leaderless group situational technique places each candidate in a role playing situation within the group context. The candidate must promote or "champion" a specific idea or staff member for promotion. How the candidate presents the case is assessed for signs of assertiveness, energy, expository skill, or other defined characteristics of leadership.

3. The case analysis technique presents the candidate with background information on a specific organizational problem such as a financial analysis case. The candidate is asked to prepare his/her recommendations for handling or resolving the problem.

4. Information-seeking exercises provide a candidate with basic information regarding a specific problem. The candidate is allowed access to a resource for addressing questions about the problem within a set time frame in order to analyze the problem in light of the newly acquired information and make recommendations for its resolution.

5. The in-basket test is a rather elaborate, realistic situational test that simulates certain aspects of an administrator's paper work. It consists of facsimiles of the letters, memoranda, staff studies and other contents of the in-basket as is found on every administrator's desk. Each candidate is provided with pencils, paper, memo pads, calendar, letterheads, and other appropriate office material and is instructed to respond to in-basket items as if actually on the job.

These different types of situational tests provide excellent formats for developing new approaches to laboratory training experiences emphasizing simulated exercises. While the simulator model of training has been used successfully in training airplane pilots, it is only in recent years that simulations have been developed for training people in industry, education, and the human services.

Simulation design and implementation also serve as a much needed forum for bringing together management tasks, the needs of the learner, and the results of prior research. This process serves as the foundation for the development of specific learning objectives that can be measured when the learner completes a simulation experience. Measuring the learner's knowledge and skills applied to a specific situation should open up new approaches to the evaluation of management training.

Simulations that incorporate the techniques of role playing, in-basket, and leaderless groups provide the participant with an opportunity to learn from peers through shared experiences. In addition, participants learn from the instructor through the debriefing process in which theoretical concepts are applied to simulated experiences. Participants also are able to experience risk-taking, an opportunity that occurs only rarely in courses or internships. They also gain exposure to a wide variety of problem definitions and strategies for solutions. Through increasingly more refined management knowledge and skills derived from dealing with progressively more complex situations, participants have a unique opportunity to link theory with practice.

SIMULATIONS AS LEARNING TOOLS

A simulation is a series of exercises based on a theme which reflects current and projected realities of agency operations. The simulation serves as a bridge between classroom learning and field experience. Simulations provide participants with an opportunity to develop new skills and gain new knowledge about the administrative aspects of agency operation. The participant in a simulation is led to project him/herself into real life situations based on the use of specific concepts and/or facts which have been presented. Thus, a simulation's purpose is to increase both the participant's level of functioning and the participant's mastery of content; to make connections between theoretical constructs and the complexities of agency life.

Simulations are based on models of reality, not necessarily upon reality itself (Lauffer, 1973). This allows for more inclusion of theoretical constructs and an emphasis on "things as they should be" as well as "things as they are." The utility of this feature of simulations is that any one simulation is equally valid and useful for both current and future practitioners. For participants who lack agency experience, a simulation offers the chance to convert knowledge into action, to try many different models of action to discover what is best suited to their personalities, and to gain experience with practical simulated situations. For practitioners, or those already in the field, a simulation offers the chance to develop conceptual "handles" that will increase their understanding of their work, to experiment safely with new methods and processes, and to introduce new or reinforce old cognitive and affective learning.

Simulations can be used for three purposes: for teaching and learning; for research or data gathering; and for social or interpersonal intervention (Lauffer, 1973). Simulations are most commonly used for teaching and learning in a university and continuing education setting. These management simulations for mental health and human service administration were designed primarily for teaching and learning experiences.

One of the overall goals of simulations is to shape behavior, not into a standard mold but into demonstrated skillful analyzing and problem-solving behaviors. The direction in which participants' behavior will be shaped is a question of administrative philosophy in which a clear-cut choice must be made. Argyris and Schon (1974) have attempted to define the skills and learning situations required to increase the effectiveness of professional administrators seeking competence in skills such as planning, communicating, and negotiating. These skills have been identified as theories of action by Argyris and Schon (1974) who have developed Model I and Model II theories. This series of simulations attempts to shape behavior of participants toward the end of Model II.

MODEL I - From research observations of ineffective administrative practice, Argyris and Schon define four governing variables which characterize the professional behavior of most administrators: (1) defining goals and trying to achieve them; (2) maximizing winning and minimizing losing; (3) minimizing the generation or expression of negative feelings; and (4) being rational. The action strategies or intervention methods used by administrators to operationalize these variables are identified as: (1) designing and managing their organizational environments unilaterally; (2) owning and controlling their tasks; (3) unilaterally protecting self; and (4) unilaterally protecting others. If the individual administrator adopts any of these four action strategies, he/she seeks to control others and resists being influenced by others. If an individual resists being controlled, certain consequences follow: (1) individuals will be defensive; (2) interpersonal and group relationships will be more defensive than facilitative; (3) defensiveness in individual and interpersonal relations will generate group norms which support this behavior (norms such as conformity, antagonism, and mistrust); and (4) there will be little freedom to explore new alternatives.

MODEL II - In contrast to the variables and strategies of Model I, Model II reflects increased intervention effectiveness, growth, and learning. The governing variables of Model II are: (1) maximizing valid information; (2) maximizing free and informed choice; and (3) maximizing internal commitments to decisions made. The resulting action strategies or intervention methods used by administrators to operationalize Model II governing variables are: (1) making decisions and managing the environment as a shared task; (2) making protection of self or others a joint project; and (3) speaking in directly observable categories. One of the consequences of Model II behavior is encouraging open, facilitative, and minimally defensive behavior. Model II reduces defensiveness in interpersonal and group relationships and encourages open discussion, helping behavior, and free expression of new or risky ideas. Group norms will move toward growth and new learning with trust, individuality, power sharing, and cooperation as standards. As individuals achieve more psychological success, they display greater self-awareness and acceptance, which leads to providing more valid information. In sum, Model II facilitates the learning of others, which in turn facilitates one's own learning.

The actual shaping process used in these simulations follows three steps. The first step is to provide some type of evaluative instrument

or exercise which will enable the participant to gain a clear picture
of his/her present behavior. The second step is to encourage the
participant to experiment with new ways of behaving through role play
or comparing his/her behavior with other participants' behavior and
providing a model. The third step is to reinforce either the new
behavior and/or the model through feedback and debriefings.

In attempting to encourage the development of Model II behavior
among participants, five basic issues were identified as critical in
the process of designing these simulations: (1) the development of
learning objectives; (2) simulations and the learning process;
(3) simulation and participant anxiety; (4) simulation realism; and
(5) simulation and learning outcomes.

LEARNING OBJECTIVES - Learning objectives for simulations should
be specific and related to the target audience. The designer should be
clear about the knowledge, skills, and values he/she wishes to teach
and the learning needs of the potential participants. In this series
of simulations, each simulation has one overall goal and several
enabling objectives. The goal speaks to the entire simulation; the
enabling objectives, to the different frames. These statements of
goal and enabling objectives should serve as criteria by which each
participant can evaluate his/her own learning.

SIMULATION AND THE LEARNING PROCESS - Three important principles
of learning are reinforcement, effect, and intensity. Reinforcement is
provided in these simulations through debriefing. Reinforcement is not
always immediate, however, as this reflects reality. The simulation is
purposefully kept fairly simple, so that the participant can see the
effect of his/her actions. Complex situations are divided into
manageable learning segments and the participant is taken through the
situations one step at a time. Intensity is thus reduced to provide
more realistic demands upon the participant's cognitive and affective
abilities. This, in turn, helps to decrease participant anxiety.

SIMULATION AND PARTICIPANT ANXIETY - To some degree, all learning
creates stresses, tensions, and frustrations for the learner. This is
also true of simulations, particularly for those participants who are
not accustomed to experiential training. Stress on the participant can
result from an information underload (boredom), or emphasis on

competition. It is important that stress and participant's anxiety be kept at a level which is not dysfunctional to the simulation. Some anxiety can lead to productive learning. Instructors who are able to share their own doubts and anxieties can help the participants confront their own anxieties.

SIMULATION REALISM - Realism encourages spontaneous participant involvement in the simulation, minimizes the projection of frustration onto the training situation, and maintains the level of participant involvement needed to encourage participants to experiment with various approaches to problem solving. Credibility is highly important; the simulation should promote clarity and not necessarily the designer's own point of view.

SIMULATION AND LEARNING OUTCOMES - The impressions which participants gain from participation in simulations are at least as lasting as are the facts which are presented. Accordingly, it is important that participants be encouraged to discuss the formal model or assumptions upon which a simulation is based. Participants should recognize that simulations may represent an altered view of reality. If a simulation has excluded certain constraints or limitations, the debriefing should include discussion of these factors. The real problem is that of achieving a proper balance between the simplicity and complexity of administrative practice.

As stated before, simulations are a middle ground between didactic and experiential learning and commonly include both, alternating between reading-comprehension and acting-evaluation. Each serves to clarify the other. They also resemble programmed instruction in that simulations can be a completely self-contained package of instruction which does not require any other material to impart its content. Simulations also include immediate feedback, though often times much of this feedback is self-generated. Some participants may want to form diads or triads to debrief simulations informally over coffee.

Unlike most programmed instruction, simulations involve interacting with other persons--using other persons as sources of knowledge such as fellow learners, partners, groups, or instructors. Unlike a traditional classroom setting, simulations require both collaboration and cooperation, both individual and group work. Unlike most workshops, it is almost impossible for any one participant to sit through a simulation and not participate. There are questions that must be answered, roles that must be played, exercises that must be completed. Thus, a simulation serves as a trigger mechanism by encouraging participants to become actively involved in doing and learning.

All the simulations are designed to help the participant become a better member of a small, task-oriented group. Most administrators spend a great deal of time working with small groups of people, trying to produce a product as the result of their collective work such as a new program, improved staff morale, next year's budget, etc. These simulations point out specific behaviors which are functional and dysfunctional to a task-oriented group and provide models, both experiential and conceptual, for the participant.

The success of simulations in management training is based on the ability of participants to relax and play with a new approach to learning. Future success also will require a new alliance between practicing human service administrators and educators teaching in administration programs. This alliance is predicated on the ability of educators to move beyond the classroom and on the ability of administrators to move beyond day-to-day crises to help with conceptualizing the ingredients of effective management. The challenge for both educators and administrators is to equip future administrators with the knowledge, skills, and values necessary for managing the multiple demands inherent in a changing human service industry.

ACKNOWLEDGMENTS

Many people assisted with the development of these simulations. First, I want to express my appreciation to the National Institute of Mental Health, Social Work Training Branch (especially Dr. Nelson Smith and Dr. Milton Wittman) who made it possible to explore new territory while preparing social workers for careers in mental health administration. Second, I want to acknowledge the support and encouragement which I received from Dean Diane Bernard, Florida State University School of Social Work, throughout the three years of the experimental training project. Third, I am grateful to my colleagues Dr. Patricia Y. Martin, Ms. Lyn Davis, Ms. Beth G. Sodec, and Mr. John Whiddon who each contributed immeasurably to the development of the simulations. I also want to thank Carl Reine, University of Michigan at Flint whose thinking laid the groundwork for the Maxras simulation. Special thanks also goes to Ms. Lyn Davis who did an outstanding job of editing the simulations and who co-authored the Instructor's Guide which accompanies this book. In addition, our two consultants, Dr. Armand Lauffer (University of Michigan) and Mr. George Drain (Human Systems, Inc.) made important contributions to the development and refinement of the simulations. And last, but definitely not least, I want to express my appreciation to three outstanding secretaries, Mrs. Sandy Brown, Mrs. Ivy Oliveros, and Mrs. Diane Stutzman, who patiently and diligently typed and retyped many of the pages you are about to read.

REFERENCES

Anderson, W. F., Frieden, B. J., & Murphy, M. J. Managing human services. Washington, D. C.: International City Management Association, 1977.

Argyris, C., & Schon, D. C. Theory in practice: Increasing professional effectiveness. San Francisco: Jossey-Bass, 1974.

Ehlers, W. H., Austin, M. J., & Prothero, J. C. Administration for the human services: An introductory programmed text. New York: Harper and Row, 1976.

Feldman, S. (Ed.). The administration of mental health services. Springfield, Ill.: Charles C Thomas, 1973.

Hasenfeld, Y., & English, R. A. (Eds.). Human service organizations. Ann Arbor, Mich.: The University of Michigan Press, 1974.

Lauffer, A. The aim of the game. Ann Arbor, Mich.: Gamed Simulations, Inc., 1973.

Slavin, S. (Ed.). Social administration: The management of the social services. New York: The Haworth Press, 1978.

1

VALUES AND ETHICS

I. PURPOSE

In order to function as an effective human service administrator, one needs to be fully aware of one's own personal values, professional values, and personal management philosophy. "Values and Ethics" is designed to help participants clarify those values. A secondary purpose of this simulation is to increase participants' skill in, and appreciation of the importance of, functioning in task-oriented groups.

This simulation serves as the introductory exercise in a series of exercises designed to increase the knowledge and skills required of a human services administrator.

II. GOALS AND ENABLING OBJECTIVES

Goals:

1. To clarify one's working set of values and ethics in human service administration.

2. To improve one's functioning as a member of a task-oriented group.

Enabling Objectives:

1. To acquire an understanding of one's views of critical issues and personal management philosophy through personally derived data on self-perceptions.

2. To engage in a process of value and ethics clarification in order to derive a personal set of managerial ethics.

3. To compare data from peers, gathered from an exercise in group process assessment, with data from one's own self-perceptions; to gain insights about one's managerial behavior and style of working in a group.

III. PROCEDURES

FRAME I - Self-Assessment

     Step 1. Managerial Philosophies for the Human Services
           (15 minutes)
     Step 2. Debriefing Managerial Philosophies (5 minutes)
     Step 3. Goals for Learning Group Process Skills (10 minutes)
     Step 4. Debriefing Goals for Learning Group Process Skills
           (20 minutes)

FRAME II - Value Conflicts

     Step 1. Prioritizing Values (10 minutes)
     Step 2. Presentation of Individual Rankings (5 minutes)
     Step 3. Developing Administrative Implications (15 minutes)
     Step 4. Debriefing (10 minutes)

FRAME III - Building a Managerial Code of Ethics

     Step 1. Group Task Work and Observation on Ethics (30 minutes)
     Step 2. Reversal of Group Roles (30 minutes)
     Step 3. Feedback on Observation Chart (10 minutes)
     Step 4. Debriefing (10 minutes)

FRAME IV - Group Process Analysis

     Step 1. "Group Process Analysis" (20 minutes)
     Step 2. Evaluation of Individual Self-Awareness (10 minutes)
     Step 3. Debriefing (15 minutes)

FRAME I

SELF-ASSESSMENT

Everyone spends some time in the course of their daily work evaluating themselves in the light of work situations and interpersonal relationships. The objective of this frame is to focus attention on the identification and assessment of each participant's "managerial self." While it is difficult to separate one's personal uniqueness from one's managerial qualities, it is important to develop an approach to self-assessment which provides the individual with tools for periodic evaluation. The importance of self-assessment is the conscious commitment to evaluate oneself over time in terms of managerial effectiveness in the area of interpersonal relations. Obviously there are other important areas for evaluation (e.g., Did your request for a budget increase actually get approved? Did you actually gain a new staff member for your unit?, etc.).

This frame focuses on two approaches to managerial self-assessment. The first step includes an inventory for assessing one's managerial philosophy based on McGregor's (1971) concepts of how managers and supervisors motivate others in the context of organizational life. The second step includes an inventory on group process skills designed to organize one's perceptions of communication, observation, self-disclosure, tolerance for emotional situations, and social relationships. These are not tests in that there is no way to pass or fail. The results of these self-assessment inventories are for personal use only. The insights gained from these inventories should prove to be useful outcomes of this simulation.

Step 1. Managerial Philosophies for the Human Services (15 minutes)

On the following pages are 18 statements relating to managerial philosophy. After reading each statement, decide how much you agree or disagree with each statement or indicate if you are uncertain. Circle the number after each statement that best indicates your reaction to that statement.

MANAGERIAL PHILOSOPHIES FOR THE HUMAN SERVICES

		I AGREE			uncertain	I DISAGREE		
		very much	on the whole	a little	uncertain	a little	on the whole	very much
If at all possible, the average human service worker will avoid work.	#	7	6	5	4	3	2	1
Using authority to direct workers is the best way for a human service manager to get work done.	#	7	6	5	4	3	2	1
Eliminating emotionality and striving for rationality are the hallmarks of a good human service administrator.	#	7	6	5	4	3	2	1
The reason most agency employees work is because they have to.	#	7	6	5	4	3	2	1
The average human service worker is able to handle a certain amount of autonomy and independence on the job.	*	7	6	5	4	3	2	1
"The greatest amount of reward for the least effort" is the motto of most human service workers.	#	7	6	5	4	3	2	1
Human service managers can usually trust their subordinates.	*	7	6	5	4	3	2	1
Rather than take initiative, most workers prefer to be directed.	#	7	6	5	4	3	2	1
If human service supervisors did not control and direct their subordinates, work toward the agency's goal would never get done.	#	7	6	5	4	3	2	1
More than anything else, the average human service worker wants security.	#	7	6	5	4	3	2	1
Under the right conditions, the average human service worker will learn not only to accept but also to seek responsibility.	*	7	6	5	4	3	2	1

		I AGREE				I DISAGREE		
		very much	on the whole	a little	uncertain	a little	on the whole	very much
For many tasks, the worker's inner self-control will eliminate the manager's need to control the worker.	*	7	6	5	4	3	2	1
A worker who is a self-starter is fairly rare in any human service agency.	#	7	6	5	4	3	2	1
In dealing with organizational problems, most workers display a fairly high degree of imagination, ingenuity, and creativity.	*	7	6	5	4	3	2	1
Motivation through money and fringe benefits is the only way to make sure a worker is productive.	#	7	6	5	4	3	2	1
Trusting one's peers and colleagues in most agencies is natural and right.	*	7	6	5	4	3	2	1
When faced with potential conflict, a manager's best response is to "divide and conquer" by encouraging communication between subordinates and one's self and discouraging communication among subordinates.	#	7	6	5	4	3	2	1
Most workers will not work toward human service agency goals unless they are coerced, controlled, or directed.	#	7	6	5	4	3	2	1

When you have read each statement and circled your response for each statement, total the point values for all the statements that have a "#" between the statement and the response. Enter this total in the appropriate space on the "Tally Sheet." Now do the same procedure for the "*" statements.

Tally Sheet

Managerial Philosophies for Human Services

Total for items noted by an # _____ -- Theory X

Interpretation

        High acceptance of Theory X   -- 56 to 84

        Medium acceptance of Theory X -- 26 to 55

        Low acceptance of Theory X   -- 12 to 25

Total for items noted by an * _____ -- Theory Y

Interpretation

        High acceptance of Theory Y   -- 38 to 42

        Medium acceptance of Theory Y -- 28 to 37

        Low acceptance of Theory Y   -- 6 to 27

The interpretation of the tally scores have been made for training purposes only and therefore no assumptions have been made about their validity or reliability across populations of participants.

Step 2. Debriefing Managerial Philosophies (5 minutes)

Turn back to the "Tally Sheet" and look at the two scores you noted in the blanks for "#" and "*" to see which theory plays a more important part for you in management. Listed below are the definitions of Theory X and Theory Y.

THEORY X

1. Work is inherently distasteful to the average human service worker.
2. Workers have little desire for responsibility, are not ambitious, and prefer direction.
3. Workers have low capacities for creativity in solving human service agency problems.
4. Workers are motivated by "creature comfort" and security comforts.
5. Staff work toward the agency's objectives and goals only if they are coerced and closely controlled.

THEORY Y

1. The expenditure of physical and mental effort in work is as natural as play or rest.
2. Workers will exercise self-direction and self-control in the service of objectives to which they are committed. External control and the threat of punishment are ineffective means for generating either commitment or effort toward agency objectives.
3. Workers' commitments to an objective is a function of the intrinsic rewards associated with delivering human services.
4. The average worker learns, under proper conditions, not only to accept but to seek responsibility.
5. The capacity to exercise a relatively high degree of imagination, ingenuity, and creativity in the solution of human service agency problems is widely, not narrowly, distributed in the population of workers.

Most managers ascribe to Theory X. But most research in motivation and social psychology affirms that Theory Y speaks to the manner in which people truly are motivated. In other words, Theory X tends to be most managers' perceptions of the world, but Theory Y tends to be the reality of the world. What was the relationship between your Theory X and Theory Y scores? If one score is in a higher range than the other, then you tend to accept the theory with the higher score more than the other theory. If the scores are in the same range, then you reflect a balanced orientation to Theory X and Theory Y. Do these interpretations confirm your prior perceptions of yourself or do they differ?

Step 3. Goals for Learning Group Process Skills (10 minutes)

On the following pages are 48 statements related to group process skills (adapted from Resnick, 1978). Since all managers work with individuals and groups, it is important to monitor one's group process skills over time. Needless to say, this monitoring is a lifelong process in which all of us seek to improve our capabilities in dealing effectively with the ongoing processes reflected in the life of any group (e.g., staff group, community group, advisory group, etc.).

The following inventory provides an opportunity to reassess one's goals for developing and improving group process skills. After each statement is reviewed, there are three responses which need to be evaluated so that one response can be marked (X): doing all right; need to do it more; need to do it less. At the end of each section in the inventory is a space for the inclusion of an additional skill. Feel free to add your own skill area.

After completing the inventory, review the responses and circle three or four of the statements which could serve as personal goals for your participation in simulations like this one.

GOALS FOR LEARNING GROUP PROCESS SKILLS

COMMUNICATION SKILLS	Doing all right	Need to do it more	Need to do it less
1. Amount of talking in group			
2. Being brief and concise			
3. Being forceful			
4. Drawing others out			
5. Listening alertly			
6. Thinking before I talk			
7. Keeping my remarks on the topic			
8. _____			

OBSERVATION SKILLS

	Doing all right	Need to do it more	Need to do it less
9. Noting tension in the group			
10. Noting who talks to whom			
11. Noting interest level of group			
12. Sensing feelings of individuals			
13. Noting who is being "left out"			
14. Noting reaction to my comments			
15. Noting when group avoids a topic			
16. _____			

SELF-DISCLOSURE

	Doing all right	Need to do it more	Need to do it less
17. Telling others what I feel			
18. Hiding my emotions			
19. Disagreeing openly			
20. Expressing warm feelings			
21. Expressing gratitude			
22. Being humorous			
23. Being angry			
24. _____			

TOLERANCE FOR EMOTIONAL SITUATIONS	Doing all right	Need to do it more	Need to do it less
25. Being able to face conflict/anger			
26. Being able to face closeness and affection			
27. Being able to face disappointment			
28. Being able to stand silence			
29. Being able to stand tension			
30. _____			

SOCIAL RELATIONSHIPS

31. Competing to outdo others			
32. Acting dominant toward others			
33. Trusting others			
34. Being helpful			
35. Being protective			
36. Calling attention to one's self			
37. Being able to stand up for myself			
38. Ability to be open with others			
39. _____			

GENERAL

40. Understanding why I do what I do (insight)			
41. Encouraging comments on my own behavior (feedback)			
42. Accepting help willingly			
43. Making my mind up firmly			
44. Criticizing myself			
45. Waiting patiently			
46. Allowing myself to have fun			
47. Allowing myself time alone			
48. _____			

Step 4. Debriefing Goals for Learning Group Process Skills
   (20 minutes)

The first step in debriefing your goals is to share the three or four statements which you circled on the inventory with another person (10 minutes). You are free to choose the other person from among all the simulation participants but the easiest approach may be the selection of the person sitting immediately to your right or left. This brief sharing process is designed to give everyone an opportunity to share part of their assessment in order to clarify their goals verbally and to engage in shared learning. This experience is designed to be brief so it is important not to engage in an analysis of each other. When the entire simulation is completed, you may want to meet privately with your partner again (e.g., over coffee or lunch) to share your perceptions on how much progress each one of you has made toward the achievement of your goals.

The second step in the debriefing process (10 minutes) is to participate with the instructor and all the other simulation participants in answering the following questions:

1. Are the statements in this inventory on goals for learning group process skills realistic?

2. Are there statements which were left out and should be added?

3. Was the sharing of your goals with a partner uncomfortable?

4. How much self-disclosure is useful for managers and supervisors to make with superiors and subordinates?

5. Are there cultural differences which result in different group process communication patterns reflected by members of different minority groups?

FRAME II

VALUE CONFLICTS

While the previous frame emphasized group process skills and managerial philosophy, this frame focuses more specifically on clarifying values which affect your managerial perspective. Clarifying values is an important process for the development of a managerial self-concept. Equally important are the ethics which govern managerial behavior and this issue will be addressed in the frame that follows this one.

Step 1. Prioritizing Values (10 minutes)

In the space provided below, rank the three values in each category according to your beliefs or according to their importance to you. Rank them in order of importance--the most important first, the next in order of importance second, and so on. You will have 10 minutes to complete this part of the exercise. Work on your own without talking to others in the group.

PATIENTS

_____ A. Violent people should be locked up in mental hospitals.

_____ B. Diagnostic labeling of patients should be eliminated since it infringes on the civil rights of people.

_____ C. Treating the whole family should take precedence over treating individuals.

STAFF

_____ A. Mental health professionals (psychiatrist, psychologist, social worker, nurse, etc.) in a mental health center should be able to function without any supervision.

_____ B. Staff should determine who gets served by a mental health center based only on the susceptibility of symptoms to successful treatment (e.g., "creaming").

_____ C. All staff with clinical competence should continue to assume responsibilities for some patients when they perform full-time administrative duties.

EXECUTIVE

_____A. Mental health center directors should always seek
            multiple sources of funding.

_____B. The director of a mental health center should be a
            physician if the needs of patients and the community
            are to be met.

_____C. The architecture of a mental health facility should
            reflect the needs and procedures of the mental health
            program.

After all participants have ranked their value preferences, move
on to Step 2.

Step 2. Presentation of Individual Rankings (5 minutes)

For this, and the next step in this exercise, all participants
should be subdivided into an even number of subgroups of three
to six members each. Once the small groups are formed, each group
member is to share the one most important value related to each
category of patients, staff, and the executive. Please note that this
is not the time to discuss in depth the various statements made or to
explore the relative merits of group members' statements. Rather, it
is a time for each group member to express and articulate his or her
rankings. Other group members should feel free to ask for
clarification and explanation, if necessary, but should essentially
listen to, and try to understand, what others are expressing.

Every group member should have time to read aloud and clarify
their rankings. Note below the value statement for each category which
received the most support from the group members.

PATIENTS	STAFF	EXECUTIVE
Statement A _____	Statement A _____	Statement A _____
Statement B _____	Statement B _____	Statement B _____
Statement C _____	Statement C _____	Statement C _____

After your group has finished this step, please move on to
Step 3.

Step 3. Developing Administrative Implications (15 minutes)

Ranking the value statements in Step 1 should have been difficult because those value statements reflect complex problems that are not easily prioritized. Perhaps you felt you were choosing the least of the three evils. Listening to the priority ranking of other participants might have confirmed your opinion about the complexity of the underlying themes of these value statements as well as the diverse ways in which people attempt to deal with them.

In this step, you and your group will have the opportunity to develop three administrative implications (e.g., impact on the operation of the agency) for each of the value statements which received the most support from the group members as a whole. Work as a group for the next ten minutes and note at least three implications which derive from your group's top three statements on patients, staff, and executive.

ADMINISTRATIVE IMPLICATIONS REGARDING VALUE STATEMENT WHICH
RECEIVED THE MOST SUPPORT RELATED TO PATIENTS

1. _____

_____

2. _____

_____

3. _____

_____

ADMINISTRATIVE IMPLICATIONS REGARDING VALUE STATEMENT WHICH
RECEIVED THE MOST SUPPORT RELATED TO STAFF

1. _____

_____

2. _____

_____

3. _____

_____

ADMINISTRATIVE IMPLICATIONS REGARDING VALUE STATEMENT WHICH
RECEIVED THE MOST SUPPORT RELATED TO <u>EXECUTIVES</u>

1. _____

    _____

2. _____

    _____

3. _____

    _____

When your group has finished this step, proceed to Step 4.

Step 4. Debriefing (10 minutes)

Within your group, answer the following questions:

1. How much difficulty did your group experience in developing
   administrative implications? Was consensus easily achieved?
   If so, why? If not, why not?

2. Turn back for a moment to your scores on the Managerial
   Philosophies Inventory in Frame I. What is the relationship
   between your management philosophy and your perspectives on
   values?

3. Values are generally broad statements involving attitudes and
   beliefs. How much does the situation in which you are working
   affect your commitment to values which permeate the human
   services?

FRAME III

BUILDING A MANAGERIAL CODE OF ETHICS

In the previous frame, participants worked with value statements in an effort to clarify their own values. If values relate primarily to beliefs and attitudes, then ethics relate more to one's own behavior. Ethics serve as the guidelines for one's practice. In this frame, participants will work toward clarifying their own set of ethics.

Step 1. Group Task Work and Observation on Ethics (30 minutes)

Each small group should find one other small group with whom they will work. Make sure that the groups are separated from one another so that disturbance will be minimal. Decide which of the two groups will go first. This group will be the work group. The other group will become the observation group.

TASK OF THE WORK GROUP - The first step is for each member to work separately and rank the students in the hypothetical code of ethics for human service administrators found on the following page. Take no more than 10 minutes to rank these statements on your own. As soon as all members have finished working individually, move right on into the second part where you will work together, for at least 20 minutes, to develop a ranking which reflects the group's consensus. Group discussion and work, therefore, should be toward developing a composite group ranking of ethics.

TASK OF THE OBSERVATION GROUP - While the members of the work group are working individually, read the hypothetical code of ethics found on the following page. Review the observation chart which follows the Code of Ethics. When the members of the work group begin to develop a ranking that reflects the group's opinion on the hypothetical code of ethics, work by yourself and observe the behavior of the members of the work group and the group as a whole closely. Take whatever notes you need to fill out the observation chart. By the time the work group is finished, at the end of this step, you should have your chart filled out completely.

After 30 minutes, the groups should move on to the next step in this part of this exercise.

GROUP RANKING	INDIVIDUAL RANKING		HUMAN SERVICE ADMINISTRATOR HYPOTHETICAL CODE OF ETHICS (adapted from Immegart & Burroughs, 1970)
_____	_____	A.	The professional administrator constantly upholds the honor and dignity of his/her profession in all actions and relations with clients, colleagues, board members, and the public.
_____	_____	B.	The professional administrator obeys local, state, and national laws, holds himself/herself to high ethical and moral standards, and gives loyalty to his/her country and to the cause of democracy and liberty.
_____	_____	C.	The professional administrator accepts the responsibility throughout his/her career to master and to contribute to the growing body of specialized knowledge, concepts, and skills which characterize his/her profession.
_____	_____	D.	The professional administrator strives to provide the finest possible services to all persons in a city, county, state, or country.
_____	_____	E.	The professional administrator applying for a position or entering into contractual agreement seeks to preserve and enhance the prestige and status of his/her profession.
_____	_____	F.	The professional administrator carries out in good faith policies duly adopted by a board of directors or legislative body and the regulations of state authorities and renders professional service to the best of his/her ability.
_____	_____	G.	The professional administrator honors the public trust of his/her position above any economic or social rewards.
_____	_____	H.	The professional administrator does not permit consideration of private gain nor personal economic interest to affect the discharge of his/her professional responsibilities.

OBSERVATION CHART ON GROUP PROCESS

1. Did the group seem to develop a plan to deal with the task? _____
   (Took easier items first, difficult items last; high priority vs.
   low priority items; seemed to have no plan.) If so, what was it?

   _____

   _____

2. How much freedom was there to express ideas in the group?
   (Check one)

   Great amount [ ]   Moderate amount [ ]   Hardly any at all [ ]

3. How much interest was there in completing the task?

   Great amount [ ]   Moderate amount [ ]   Hardly any at all [ ]

4. Were there group members who contributed to getting the task done?
   If so, who?

   _____

5. If strong disagreements emerged in the group, who worked to settle
   them?

   _____

6. Assume that the time the group spent working as a group totals
   100%. What percentage of this 100% did the group devote to task
   completion, and what percentage to group maintenance? (Task
   completion refers to working on the rankings to be assigned to
   each item. Group maintenance refers to time spent settling
   conflicts, involving marginal members of the group, or making sure
   that members of the group do not become alienated.)

   _____%_____ + _____%_____ = 100%
   Percentage of time spent   Percentage of time spent
   on task completion   on group maintenance

Step 2. Reversal of Group Roles (30 minutes)

The roles of all groups should now be reversed. The observation group becomes the work group and sits in the center, and the work group becomes the observation group. For the next 30 minutes, Step 1 of this frame is repeated with each group assuming the other group's roles as set forth in Step 1. After 30 minutes all groups should be ready to move on to the next step, Step 3.

Step 3. Feedback on Observation Chart (10 minutes)

The instructor should select two members from each group (since both groups have now completed the observation chart) to provide feedback according to the items on the observation chart. Begin with the second observation group or the group which just finished completing the observation chart.

Step 4. Debriefing (10 minutes)

Now return to your work group and discuss the following questions:

1. Does the hypothetical code of ethics represent a code to which you could adhere? Why?

2. If your group could develop its own code, what would be its major components?

3. Do you see a need for a managerial code of ethics in the human services? Why or why not?

FRAME IV

GROUP PROCESS ANALYSIS

For this frame, you and your work group from the preceding frame should sit together. It will help if your work group sits a bit apart from the other work groups, so that their conversations will not disturb your group.

Step 1. "Group Process Analysis" (20 minutes)

The final exercise in this simulation will assess the contributions of individuals to the group process. Your assessment of your peers will be conveyed to them anonymously. Confine your assessments only to the work group in which you participated in the last frame. Include all the time that you functioned as a group, from the beginning of the simulation.

The first step in assessment is to write the names of all the members of your group, including yourself, on the form found later in this step entitled "Assessment of All Group Members." Put your name at the top of the list.

The second step is to rank-order the members of the group according to the degree of influence each had upon the functioning of the group. Include yourself in this ranking. Use "1" for "most influence" and lower numbers for less influence. Use only as many numbers as you have group members. (For example, if your group has five members, do not rank anyone lower than 5.) Do not agonize over your choices; just make the choices quickly and write the number in the appropriate space next to the name.

The third step involves the Description Items which appear on the page following the assessment form. You will be applying these items to yourself and to your fellow group members, but, for now, simply read the Description Items. When you have finished reading the Description Items, choose at least three but no more than six of these items that apply to each member of your group, including yourself. Start with yourself and then move on to the other group members, recording the letters for each item on the form entitled "Assessment of All Group

Members." When choosing Description Items for each member, be as honest and as objective as you can.

When each member has completed the "Assessment of All Group Members" form, copy on a separate sheet of paper your name and the headings for description items and rank. See the page following the list of Description Items for an example. Place your name at the top, and place this sheet where all members of your group have access to it (in the center of your group). When someone else has placed his/her sheet in the center, take that sheet and copy the Influence Rank and Description Items which you gave that person from your list. When you have finished copying your ratings for that person, return the sheet to the center and pick up another person's sheet and mark his/hers as you did the first sheet. Do not write on your own sheet. Repeat this process until you have written on all members' sheets and keep track of each member by checking off their name after you have added your Description Items to each person's sheet.

When all members have marked the sheets of all other members, retrieve your own sheet. At the bottom of your own assessment sheet, tally your Description Items and your Influence Ranks (i.e., put a mark by "A" for each "A" you received, a mark by "B" for each "B" you received, etc.). When all members of your work group have tallied their Description Items and their Influence Ranks, tell your instructor.

ASSESSMENT OF ALL GROUP MEMBERS

	Member's Name	Description Items	Ranking
1.	_____	_____	_____
2.	_____	_____	_____
3.	_____	_____	_____
4.	_____	_____	_____
5.	_____	_____	_____
6.	_____	_____	_____
7.	_____	_____	_____

DESCRIPTION ITEMS

A. Doesn't listen well; doesn't understand, or totally ignores the statement given before his/her statement.

B. Often tries to get group to clarify what the task is and how the group is going to get that task done.

C. Seems to require an expert's opinion all the time; continually conveys impression that group really isn't competent to do the task.

D. Projects impression that he/she is only one who knows what he/she is doing; has air of superior wisdom; continually refers to experience in his/her work, as if that were the final judge.

E. States opinions candidly without reservations; lets other members know where he/she stands, without being hostile or stubborn.

F. Speaks only to agree with other members' views; rarely states own views.

G. Brings up issues that are outside the group task.

H. Seems very intent on controlling and influencing the group; fights for power in the group.

I. Often summarizes what group has just done and tries to state what the group needs to do next.

J. Is overly concerned about how the group is doing; appears to be afraid of looking bad to others.

K. Often impatient with other members.

L. Appears bored with the whole thing.

M. Seems to get stuck on issues which are important only to him/her.

N. Gives support to those struggling to express themselves; concerned about everyone in the group.

O. Little or no observable involvement.

P. Tries to help group stay within time limits.

Q. Concerned both about getting the task done and about how members feel about the group.

R. _____(Develop your own description item)

ASSESSMENT OF INDIVIDUAL GROUP MEMBER

_____
Name of Group Member

Influence Rank   Description Items
_____   _____

_____

Tally of Influence Rank: Tally of Description Items:

1   5   A   E   I   M   Q

2   6   B   F   J   N   R

3   7   C   G   K   O

4   8   D   H   L   P

Step 2. Evaluation of Individual Self-Awareness (10 minutes)

Your instructor, using the Instructor's Guide, will tell you which Description Items relate to general characteristics of your brief involvement in group decision making. Write the letters the instructor will give you in the appropriate spaces below.

FACILITATION items are descriptions of those behaviors which contribute directly to the group's accomplishment of the task and how group members feel about the progress being made. Members can help the group accomplish the task by offering their own opinions, by listening carefully to others, by summarizing what the group has done and what it needs to do, and by stating what the group appears to have agreed upon. Members can help the group become more effective by eliciting reactions and feelings (e.g., angry, frustrated, pleased) and relating those feelings to the group process in order to see that all members feel they are contributing, active parts of the group.

The Facilitation Description Items are _____.

CONFLICT items are descriptions of conflict behaviors exhibited by members of the group. Conflict within a group can be positive or negative, depending on how it is handled. For example, differences of opinion can lead to a far superior work product, if they are handled productively. Interpersonal conflicts, however, generally are harmful to a group and to the group's work product. Conflict behaviors can result if a member is frustrated or is too concerned with striving for status in the group. Perceptual differences, in which each member of the group views each fact or issue differently due to that member's life experience, also can cause conflict. Again, conflicts of opinion can be helpful to a group; interpersonal conflict among members can be harmful to a group.

The Conflict Description Items are _____.

AVOIDANCE items are descriptions of members' actions which generally reflect withdrawal from group involvement. These behaviors are most debilitative to a group. Some of the causes of avoidance behaviors include feelings of fear, indifference, and/or impotence within the group. Members exhibiting these behaviors will not listen to what other members are saying, will not base their comments on what was said before, will talk about things that do not have anything to do with what the group is doing, or will worry about what others outside the group will think of what the group is doing.

The Avoidance Description Items are _____.

NEUTRAL items are descriptions of behaviors which are neither helpful nor harmful to a group. If the group is fairly large, and the time to accomplish the task is fairly short, then it is only natural that some members will not speak at all. It generally requires a bit of time for shy or uncertain members to begin to speak up, to express their own opinions. These types of group members may be just as interested in accomplishing the task as are the most vocal members.

The Neutral Description Items are _____.

Now look to see which Description Items and which numerical rankings were given to you most often by your fellow group members. See whether these Description Items are Facilitation, Conflict, Avoidance, or Neutral. Be sure to compare your peers' assessments with your own self-assessment (rank and Description Items) you made in Step 1.

Interpretation of the tally of Influence Rank is fairly obvious. You can match the tally of the Description Items with the tally of the Influence Rank to gain more information about your style of participation in this task-oriented group. For example,

A high score on Influence Rank (mostly "1" and "2") combined with several Conflict Description Items would mean that the group perceives you as having a strong, but less than positive, influence on the group.

A high score on Influence Rank combined with several Facilitation Description Items would mean that the group perceives you as a positive influence on the group both as a leader and as a member.

A low score on Influence Rank combined with several Avoidance Description Items would mean that the group perceives you as a member who contributes little to the group despite the fact that you felt quite involved.

REMEMBER: This evaluation was based on a very brief period of time. You might well function entirely differently in a longer group meeting or a meeting of people who you have known for some time. Also remember that this was a task-oriented group and not a growth, encounter, or counseling group. Only your style of participation in a task-oriented group was evaluated--not you as a person. Let this evaluation clue you into group process--including helpful behaviors, harmful behaviors, and the myriad interactions that take place in a successful task-oriented group. Take this evaluation only as a starting point for the future, not as a final judgment.

A key ingredient of one's "managerial self" is to utilize feedback by first looking at it from the distance of an "arm's length." All good managers seek feedback from a variety of sources before internalizing the information or making a decision. If you allow one type of feedback to upset you, then you have identified an important area for future work on developing your "managerial self."

Step 3. Debriefing (15 minutes)

1. How did your own perceptions of your functioning in a work group
    differ from how your colleagues saw you functioning? (Compare your
    self-ratings on the "Group Process Analysis" with the composite
    rating given you by the group.)

2. Recall what you saw when you observed the other work group. What
    similarities and differences in style of working are there between
    that group and your own work group?

3. How does your score on the "Group Process Analysis" fit with the
    group process goals you identified in Frame I?

4. What are your reactions to the components of this simulation
    (self-assessment, value conflicts, building a managerial code of
    ethics, and group process analysis)?

REFERENCES

Immegart, G. L., & Burroughs, J. M. Ethics and the school
    administrator. Danville, Ill.: Interstate, 1970.

McGregor, D. Theory Y: The integration of individual and
    organizational goals. In W. R. Lassey (Ed.), Leadership and
    social change. Iowa City, Iowa: University Associates Press,
    1971.

Resnick, H. Goals for skills learning. Seattle, Wash.: University
    of Washington School of Social Work, 1978, mimeo.

RELATED READINGS

Blake, R. R., & Mouton, J. S. People--The wellspring of organizational energy. In W. R. Lassey (Ed.), Leadership and social change. Iowa City, Iowa: University Associates Press, 1971.

Collins, B. E., & Guezkow, H. A social psychology of group processes for decision-making. New York: John Wiley and Sons, 1964.

Fiella, J., & Immegart, G. L. ED/AD/EX-Exercise 1: Values in education. Scottsville, N. Y.: Transnational Programs, 1971.

Hall, J. Process diagnostic. Conroe, Tex.: Teleometrics International, 1975.

Hall, J., Harvey, J. B., & Williams, M. Styles of management inventory. Conroe, Tex.: Teleometrics International, 1973.

Jacoby, J., & Terborg, J. Managerial philosophies scale. Conroe, Tex.: Teleometrics International, 1975.

Kluckhohn, F. R., & Strodtbeck, F. Variations in value orientations. New York: Harper and Row, 1961.

Maslow, A. (Ed.). New knowledge in human values. New York: Harper and Row, 1959.

Meininger, J. Success through transactional analysis. New York: Grosset and Dunlap, 1973.

Rokeach, M. The nature of human values. New York: The Free Press, 1973.

Schmidt, W. H. (Ed.). Organizational frontiers and human values. Belmont, Calif.: Wadsworth, 1970.

2

HANDLING CONFLICT

Lyn Davis

I. INTRODUCTION

Administrators and supervisors must be versed in many different facets of management. The specific knowledge and skills required for effective supervision of staff vary from agency to agency. But one skill that remains constant, regardless of agency structure and agency staffing pattern, is that of handling conflict. In the simulation that follows, participants will be presented with opportunities to learn how to develop strategies for dealing with conflict between supervisors and subordinates.

Within any agency, two separate sources of conflict (organizational and interpersonal) may produce disharmony. This disharmony may appear in two distinct locations (peer and hierarchical). Placing these sources and locations of conflict in juxtaposition can be reflected in the following chart:

SOURCES OF CONFLICT

LOCATIONS OF CONFLICT	Organizational	Interpersonal
Peer		
Hierarchical	XXXX	XXX

Thus, peer conflict (supervisor-supervisor, subordinate-subordinate) or hierarchical conflict (supervisor-subordinate) may result from organizational sources (authorities and responsibilities not clearly delegated) or interpersonal sources (personality clashes, inability of some persons to relate well to other persons). Within any of the squares in the chart, conflict may be typified as either positive or negative (functional or dysfunctional to the group). This simulation will deal only with conflict derived from organizational and interpersonal sources that surfaces in hierarchical relationships. Organizational and interpersonal sources of conflict will be dealt with separately in two different frames. In the real world, any given conflict often has its roots in both sources.

Conflict is inherently neither good nor bad. Conflict is also natural and will occur almost anywhere, at any time. Accordingly, this simulation is not intended to show how to remove conflict. Rather, this simulation is about managing conflict.

II. GOAL AND ENABLING OBJECTIVES

Goal:

To be able to develop strategies (appropriate for supervisory management) which will resolve superior-subordinate conflict which has sprung from both organizational and interpersonal sources.

Enabling Objectives:

1. To understand the positive and negative functions of conflict within an agency and to develop strategies to deal with conflict.

2. To develop and apply strategies that will resolve organizational conflict.

3. To develop and apply strategies that will resolve interpersonal conflict.

III. PROCEDURES

FRAME I - Developing Strategies

  Step 1. Understanding Positive and Negative Conflict (10 minutes)
  Step 2. Identifying Sources of Conflict (10 minutes)
  Step 3. Reaching Consensus (10 minutes)
  Step 4. Developing Strategies (15 minutes)
  Step 5. Group Strategies (20 minutes)
  Step 6. Debriefing (10 minutes)

FRAME II - Handling Organizational Conflict

  Step 1. Choosing Roles and Developing Alternative Strategies
     (15 minutes)
  Step 2. Developing a Main Strategy (10 minutes)
  Step 3. Reporting Main Strategies (10 minutes)
  Step 4. Analysis of Strategies and Debriefing (10 minutes)

FRAME III - Handling Interpersonal Conflict

  Step 1. Analyzing a Subordinate's Reaction (15 minutes)
  Step 2. Analyzing Nonproductive Responses (5 minutes)
  Step 3. Dealing with Defensiveness (20 minutes)
  Step 4. Dealing with Evasiveness (30 minutes)
  Step 5. Dealing with Withdrawal (25 minutes)
  Step 6. Dealing with Hostility (35 minutes)
  Step 7. Debriefing (10 minutes)

FRAME I

DEVELOPING STRATEGIES

Step 1. Understanding Positive and Negative Conflict (10 minutes)

Conflict is a common aspect of any situation in which more than one person is involved. Conflict within an agency can be positive or negative--that is, it can be functional or dysfunctional within an organization. Negative conflict is a conflict which concerns the very basis of a relationship and threatens to erode the consensus which originally bound the group together. Positive conflict is conflict which concerns less central issues and takes place within the context of consensus that exists in a group or organization.

Positive conflict can serve to strengthen an agency, particularly if more than one type of disagreement exists at any one time. All staff members may have an opinion or take a side on each issue that is in conflict, but rarely will the same staff member take the same side on each issue. Even if staff members disagree over as many as 20 or 30 issues at one time, the staff as a whole can still maintain consensus about the basic goal(s) of that agency.

Positive conflict can be illustrated schematically. In the following diagram, each line represents a conflict. The thickness of the line indicates the potential that conflict has for tearing apart the agency. As you can see, the lines point in almost every direction. One issue that may be divisive for the agency is crossed by several smaller lines. Thus, in a sense, the small conflicts help to keep any one positive conflict from becoming a divisive or negative conflict. A second analogy is that of a darned sock: the stitches are of different length and different strength, but each works to cover the hole and keep the sock together.

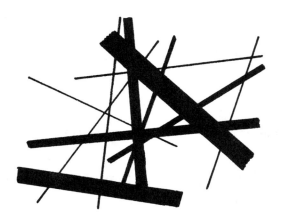

Negative conflict is a schism over one basic issue, a schism that splits the agency into two opposing camps. This is dysfunctional or harmful to an agency. Staff on either side of a negative conflict may disagree with the basic goals of the agency. Negative conflict can also be illustrated schematically. Part of the staff is on one side of the issue, and the rest of the staff is on the other side of the issue with very little, if anything, in common. The conflict is intense; there is little or no contact between sides, little or no agreement on other issues. The situation is one of "either/or," and the agency is in serious trouble.

Read each statement below and decide if it represents positive or negative conflict. Place a "P" next to each statement if it is positive conflict or an "N" if it is negative conflict.

_____ 1. Serious staff disagreement over plans for an aftercare program for released state hospital patients has led to one staff member's threatening to go to the press, "to expose the inappropriate handling of potentially dangerous people in the community." Such media coverage will probably result in loss of funding for this agency.

_____ 2. A new Mental Health Worker I position has been allocated to your agency. Much debate has been going on concerning the exact role this position should play. In addition to this debate, an argument about the "best" way for your agency to interface with other agencies has been carried on for the last few months.

_____ 3. What type of conflict is generally functional to an organization, in order to allow airing of different views on subjects that are within the basic consensus?

_____ 4. What type of conflict usually spells serious trouble for an organization, as those involved in the conflict are in two separate camps and have little contact with each other, and little in common with each other?

When you have finished placing a "P" or "N" beside each of these statements, check your answers by turning to the last page of this simulation (near the Related Readings) and then proceed to Step 2.

Step 2. Identifying Sources of Conflict (10 minutes)

As was stated in the introduction, most conflict comes from some combination of both organizational and interpersonal problems. Conflict arising from organizational sources must be treated differently from conflict arising from interpersonal sources. One source of conflict is probably very familiar to you--interpersonal relations. But what exactly causes conflict in interpersonal relations? The main culprit can be perception, or how a person views an event, a piece of data, or another person. People bring their own history with them into any situation, and thus may perceive facts differently from other people. For the purpose of this discussion, there are three common causes of interpersonal conflict:

Ideological Differences. Most of these arise from an individual's education or formal training. An example of basic ideological differences may be the different ways in which a psychiatrist, a social worker, a psychologist, a nurse, or a counselor were trained to treat a severely disturbed patient.

Personality Differences. This also includes differences in style: punctuality vs. being more flexible about time schedules; need for imposed structure vs. need for imposing one's own structure; morning persons vs. night owls.

Status Differences. Jealousy, fear, and feelings of inadequacy are the most common emotions aroused in cases where one person may have more experience than another or may hold a higher position in the agency.

There are many causes of organizational conflict which are different from the misperceptions found in interpersonal conflict. Organizational conflict seems to occur most often when changes in duties or procedures have been made or when staff wishes to make such changes. Some of the causes of organizational conflict include:

Unclear Delegation. Delegation of authority and/or responsibility is not made clear to everyone.

Inadequate Supervision. Supervisors are not exercising sufficient authority over their subordinates.

Incomplete Delegation. Responsibility has been given to a certain person for a certain task, but not the authority necessary to complete that task.

Unclear Goals or Methods for Achieving Goals. Persons working in the same unit have different measures of "success" which conflict with each other.

Now that you are familiar with the concepts of organizational and interpersonal conflict, it is time to apply that knowledge in the following situations. After reading each vignette, place an "O" for organizational or an "I" for interpersonal to indicate the source of conflict portrayed in that situation. In each situation, you are the supervisor.

_____ A. A mother has completed her intake interview in your community hospital pediatric clinic. According to the notes taken during that interview, the woman repeatedly stated, "There's nothing really wrong that I can point to and say, 'Here's my problem.' I just feel my child is too active. He's either hurting other children or himself." The staff pediatrician has prescribed medication for the youngster and told her that she should return to the clinic with her child only when she needs to have the prescription refilled. The social worker strongly disagrees with the pediatrician's treatment plan during the weekly staff meeting.

_____ B. The staffing structure of your halfway house allows for two positions for social workers: a Social Worker I and a Social Worker II. Both of these positions report directly to you. The Social Worker I has been filled for ten years by a middle-aged man who does not have a bachelor's degree in social work. The second position, Social Worker II, has experienced more turnover. Recently, it was filled by a young woman who has just completed her M.S.W. She has completed her first week of work and has made several suggestions to you about reallocation of the social workers' work load and realignment of their roles in the halfway house. Although the male social worker has been cooperating over the last six months in instituting your new procedures, he has refused to do so since the woman joined the staff. He has told you he does not want to share his office with her, even though the two social workers have traditionally worked in the same office.

_____ C. The inpatient unit of your community hospital is funded primarily on the basis of the number of patients treated each year. For example, the unit receives more money for treating two patients for one day than it receives for treating one patient for two days. You have, within the last two days, sent the forms of computation of next year's budget request to all unit heads. Today, you are sitting in the Utilization Committee's weekly staff meeting in which they discuss all suggested changes in status for their patients. The unit head wishes to discharge five patients to an extended care facility immediately, as five new patients seek admission to the already-filled unit. A staff member on the unit is arguing that these five individuals are not yet ready to be discharged. The decision on these five patients must be made by tomorrow.

_____ D. You have assigned one of your subordinates to survey your county to assess the potential number of foster parents living in this area. She reports back to you that she has been refused permission to use one of the agency's cars to conduct the survey.

_____ E. The head nurse of Ward A whom you supervise in your rehabilitation hospital believes in having a routine schedule that should be followed every day. Accordingly, she wants all patients under her care to adhere to a rather strict schedule for eating, for therapy, for recreation, for rest, etc. The head of the Recreational Therapy Unit believes that she can be most effective if she allows patients to be free to come in and leave at their own leisure, as this increases the patients' motivation. The head nurse of Ward A has sent you a memo outlining her concern: "I deliver my patients promptly to the Recreational Therapy Unit at the correct time, but my patients wander back to my ward at all hours. I feel this is disruptive to the individual patient and to my ward as a whole. The head of the Recreational Therapy Unit has, in essence, refused to comply with my requests about this matter. For the good of the patients, I feel she should be censured."

_____ F. The head child care worker for the second shift at your children's receiving home complains to you that, when his shift comes on duty, he and the other child care workers often find that the first shift workers have already left. He presents you with a list of areas that have been untended at the beginning of the second shift and the dates on which they were vacant. You check the attendance records of the first shift and find no indication of absenteeism for those dates. You ask the supervisor of the first shift if she has granted one hour's leave to any of her workers and she says that she has not.

_____ G. Part of your Public Health Division's effort to increase efficiency of referrals has been to delegate the decision to refer to all public health nurses (PHN). Accordingly, every PHN has been authorized to make referrals to the Social Services Division for fairly simple and clear-cut cases. However, they still continue to send the rest of the cases to the chief of PHNs for her to make the referrals. Formerly, the chief of PHNs had made all decisions for all referrals. The supervisor of one of the social service division units had stated in a staff meeting that he will not accept referrals unless they are from, and signed by, the chief of PHNs.

When you have finished this step, please wait for your instructor before proceeding to the next step.

<u>Step 3. Reaching Consensus</u> (10 minutes)

Divide into groups of two and compare your evaluations of each of the situations portrayed in Step 2 with each other after checking your answers with those found on this page. Do you agree with these answers? Can you see the logic behind these answers?

<u>Sources of Conflict Portrayed in Situations</u>

A. Parent and Child - Interpersonal Source. Basic ideological difference between the pediatrician and the social worker, springing from their different education and training.

B. Social Worker I and II - Interpersonal Source. Differences in status; male social worker feels jealous, perhaps fearful and inadequate, in presence of female worker.

C. Discharging Patients to Extended Care Facility - Organizational Source. Unit head and staff member have different measures of "success" that conflict with each other.

D. Foster Parents Survey - Organizational Source. Responsibility has been given to your subordinate to conduct the survey, but not the authority necessary to gain access to the tools she needs (i.e., an agency car).

E. Head Nurse and Recreational Therapy Director - Interpersonal Source. Difference in style; punctual vs. being more flexible about time schedule.

F. Child Care Worker - Organizational Source. Supervisor of first shift not exercising sufficient authority over child care workers of first shift.

G. Referral Procedures - Organizational Source. Delegation of authority and responsibility not made clear to everyone involved in the situation.

<u>Step 4. Developing Strategies</u> (15 minutes)

Although there are several alternative strategies that you can develop to meet each conflict, there are basically three general approaches that you can take. The first approach is to do nothing. The second approach is to take a hard line. The third approach is to take a soft line. These approaches apply regardless of the source or location of conflict.

Doing Nothing or Avoiding Direct Conflict

The first approach of doing nothing or avoiding direct involvement may reflect an attempt to ignore the situation, pretending that it doesn't exist. It may be a conscious or unconscious strategy for resolving conflict. The conscious decision to avoid getting involved is much more than doing nothing. Referring the matter to one of your subordinates for him/her to take care of is also different from doing nothing. Being able to choose which matters should be handled by you, the supervisor, and which matters should be handled by your subordinates requires both experience and skill. Based on the principle that conflicts are best solved closest to their origin, delegating conflict resolution to your subordinates needs to be clearly articulated so as not to leave the impression that you are doing nothing.

Hard Line

The second approach is that of taking a hard line. If you were to create a continuum that went from closed and authoritarian to open and supportive, the hard line approach would fall near the closed and authoritarian end. Please note that no value judgments are meant or implied here--open and supportive is not necessarily better than closed and authoritarian. The time to make such a judgment is during a particular situation, and that judgment will be different for each situation. When taking a hard line with conflict that arises from organizational sources, you could refer to the organizational chart of your agency and cite it as your authority from which you could make a decision and hand it down to your subordinates. When dealing with a conflict that has arisen from interpersonal sources, you could stress the importance of controlling personal feelings for the good of your agency by stressing appropriate behaviors that could be exhibited. In brief, your presence would be strongly felt during the resolution of the conflict.

Soft Line

This approach would fall on the open and supportive end of the continuum. Again, the value placed on this approach is totally dependent upon the situation. When taking a soft line in conflict that arises from organizational sources, you could shape the solution around the people involved by delegating more authority, encouraging others to respect that authority. In dealing with conflicts arising from interpersonal sources, you could elicit individual feelings about the conflict by allowing those involved in the conflict to ventilate their feelings and participate with you in the development of solutions based on open communications.

Regardless of the type of approach taken, there is no one strategy that works best for any conflict situation. Rather, you should draw up a list of all the possible alternative strategies. Such a list would undoubtedly include both hard and soft lines. From the list of alternative strategies, you would choose the strategy or combination of strategies that you think will be best for the situation. Having chosen the one strategy which you think is best, it is important to decide on what points you can be flexible, on what points you can be firm, and at what points you can switch to other strategies in your list. In other words, you should have a main strategy and one or two "fall-back" strategies.

Working in a group of six participants, select <u>one</u> of the situations in Step 2 (A through G) for everyone in the group to work on. You will be developing strategies as a group in Step 5 but, for now, work independently on the following five questions:

1. Brainstorm. Working by yourself, list all the strategies you can think of to deal with this situation. After writing down each strategy, indicate whether you think this alternative is taking a hard line or a soft line.

    _____

    _____

    _____

    _____

    _____

2. Now choose one of your alternatives, or a combination of alternatives, that you think would work best. What is it?

    _____

    _____

3. Where can you be flexible?

    _____

    _____

4. Where must you be firm?

_____

_____

5. Which alternatives are good "fall-back" strategies?

_____

_____

When all members of your group have finished this step, go on to Step 5.

Step 5. Group Strategies (20 minutes)

Begin with each member of your group reading his/her list of alternatives and the main strategy that he/she chose. Do not discuss each person's list yet. You may, however, ask questions for clarification or explanation and you should make notes on the ideas which you find most attractive.

After listening to everyone's approach, draw up one main strategy as a group dealing with your situation. Write it here:

_____

_____

_____

Choose one or two fall-back strategies. Write them here:

_____

_____

_____

_____

_____

_____

When your group has finished, you may proceed to the next step.

Step 6. Debriefing (10 minutes)

Working as an entire group, answer the following questions:

1. What problems, if any, did your group encounter in arriving at a strategy approach? Did your group develop a systematic approach while deriving a strategy? If so, what was it?

_____

_____

_____

_____

2. What would be the consequences of implementing your group's main strategy? Your group's fall-back strategies?

_____

_____

_____

_____

3. In the situation which you selected, can you identify the interpersonal conflict (ideological differences, personality differences, status differences) or organizational conflict (unclear delegation, inadequate supervision, incomplete delegation, unclear goals or methods for achieving goals)? Of all the strategies you developed (both main and fallbacks), which one was most appropriate to the specific type of conflict portrayed in your situation? Which one was least appropriate?

_____

_____

_____

_____

4. What new insights did you gain from your peers about strategy formulation for conflict resolution?

_____

_____

_____

_____

FRAME II

HANDLING ORGANIZATIONAL CONFLICT

The purpose of this frame is to increase participants' skill in handling organizational conflict. In order to accomplish this, groups of participants will work with one situation. Within this situation, roles will be assigned. Participants filling these roles will develop strategies to deal with the situation. In this way, all participants can see the benefit of considering alternative approaches to the same situation.

Step 1. Choosing Roles and Developing Alternative Strategies
 (15 minutes)

In groups of six, each participant will assume a role. Each group will be dealing with a situation which involves conflict between Betty Miles, who is Director of Social Services within a local Human Service Agency, and Jerry Silverman, who is Supervisor of Intake and Referral Services. Jerry Silverman is directly responsible to Betty Miles.

Within each small group, choose one of the following roles for each person. Make certain that each of the roles for Jerry Silverman and for Betty Miles are taken. You must fill these four roles before the organizational consultant roles are taken. The choices are:

--ego player for Betty Miles, Director of Social Services;

--alter-ego player for Betty Miles, Director of Social Services;

--ego player for Jerry Silverman, Supervisor of Intake and
  Referral Services;

--alter-ego player for Jerry Silverman, Supervisor of Intake and
  Referral Services;

--organizational consultant;

--organizational consultant

After each person has chosen a role, turn to the description of your role on the following pages and read it. Do not read anyone else's role description; read only your own. The ego and alter-ego roles should read the same description.

When all group members have finished reading their role descriptions, it is time to begin work on developing alternative strategies. Turn to the page which follows the role descriptions and note the different alternative strategies for Betty Miles and for Jerry Silverman. Those playing the roles for Betty Miles should turn to the page entitled "Alternative Strategies for Betty Miles" and work only on that page. Likewise, those playing the roles of Jerry Silverman should turn to the page entitled "Alternative Strategies for Jerry Silverman" and work only on that page. Organizational consultants should review the strategy pages for Miles and Silverman.

Work first by yourself to write down your own alternative strategies in the space provided. Do not feel that these suggested alternatives are the only feasible alternatives; they are merely suggestions to get you thinking. Feel free to choose one of the alternatives already listed or to create your own. When all members of your group have finished working individually, proceed to Step 2.

Role Description for <u>Betty Miles</u>, Director of Social Services

You are the Director of Social Services and responsible for approximately 300 social workers providing a full range of services for a medium-size community. You have been experiencing a shortage of staff, especially in providing crisis intervention services. The Supervisor of Intake and Referral (Jerry Silverman), who is directly under your supervision, was told by you over the telephone to make better utilization of his staff. In particular, he was told that the skills of the paraprofessional-level employees under his supervision must be upgraded so that social workers could be free to perform more of the professional tasks for which they are trained. He was directed to determine what training these paraprofessionals would need to upgrade their skills and then to meet with the Director of Training to work out a training program. He replied that he didn't have the time and that, in any event, the Intake and Referral Service demands extensive knowledge of the community and professional level "assessment skills" which require the use of MSWs and, at the very least, BSWs.

Note: This role description applies to both the ego and alter-ego players for Betty Miles. The ego player will decide if he/she will take a hard line or a soft line in this direction. The alter-ego player will take the opposite line from that taken by the ego player. For example, if the ego player chooses to take a hard line, then the alter-ego player must take a soft line. Decide now which line each will take.

Role Description for <u>Jerry Silverman</u>, Supervisor of Intake and Referral

You are the Supervisor of the Intake and Referral Services in a public social service agency. Of the agency's total client population for a month, two-thirds of the volume passes through Intake and Referral. The entire agency has been experiencing a shortage of staff, particularly in the Crisis Intervention Program. The Intake and Referral Unit has felt this shortage more than any other unit. In addition to that problem caused by a shortage of staff, you have not been at all pleased with the level of services given to clients by the paraprofessionals. You have come to the conclusion that paraprofessionals are fine for basic tasks but are not sufficiently skilled for the specialized intake and referral process requiring "assessment skills."

Betty Miles, who is your immediate supervisor and the Director of Social Services at the agency, telephoned you to say that the role of the paraprofessionals in your unit must be increased so that MSWs and BSWs would be freed to perform more of the professional tasks for which they were trained. You were directed specifically to determine what training the paraprofessionals would need and then work out a training program with the Director of Training. You received this phone call from Betty Miles while you were in the midst of trying to find out what really happened this morning in the Intake and Referral Unit. The harrowing incident involved a psychotic client and a paraprofessional. You told Miles that you didn't have the time and, in any event, the clients at the time of intake required professionally trained staff with extensive knowledge of community resources and professional level "assessment skills" which require the use of MSWs and, at the very least, BSWs.

Note: This role description applies to both the ego and alter-ego players for Jerry Silverman. The ego players will decide if he/she will take a hard line or a soft line in this situation. The alter-ego player will take the opposite line from that chosen by the ego player. For example, if the ego player chooses to take the hard line, then the alter-ego player must take a soft line. Decide now which one each will take.

Role Description for <u>Organizational Consultant(s)</u>

You have been on contract for the last six months to study and make recommendations about the staff of a social service agency. You are currently focusing on conflict resolution within the staff.

The Director of Social Services, Betty Miles, is responsible for 300 employees and services in a medium-size community. She has been concerned by the shortage of staff. This shortage has hit the Crisis Intervention Unit the hardest. She telephoned Jerry Silverman, who is the Supervisor of Intake and Referral Services under her direct supervision, two days ago to tell him he must make better utilization of his staff in order to release trained social workers to the Crisis Intervention Unit. In particular, he was directed to decide which skills of the paraprofessionals under his supervision needed to be upgraded and then to work with the Director of Training to develop a training program for the paraprofessionals. He replied that he didn't have the time and that, in any event, the clients at Intake and Referral required professionally trained staff with extensive knowledge of community resources and professional level "assessment skills" which require the use of BSWs and preferably MSWs.

Your job is to observe Betty Miles and Jerry Silverman as they each attempt to develop a strategy to resolve this conflict. As the ego and alter-ego players for each character work together, note which aspects of their strategies are debilitating and which are productive. Take notes, as you will be giving feedback later. You will also have the opportunity to present the strategy that you feel would be most productive for each of the characters. This strategy does not need to be one that any of the players mentioned: you may create your own. Turn to the next page and develop your own perspective on the options open to both Betty Miles and Jerry Silverman.

Alternative Strategies for Betty Miles

--Send a memo to Jerry Silverman reminding him of his obligation, with no copies to anyone.

--Send a memo to Jerry Silverman reminding him of his obligation, with copies to the following persons:

_____	_____
_____	_____
_____	_____

--Send a memo to your superior with a copy to Jerry Silverman.

--Send a memo to Jerry Silverman requesting a progress report, with no copies to anyone.

--Send a memo to Jerry Silverman requesting a progress report, with copies to the following persons:

_____	_____
_____	_____
_____	_____

--Call Jerry Silverman and request an early appointment to discuss the situation.

--Go to Jerry Silverman immediately and discuss the situation.

--Call Jerry Silverman and ask that he come to your office immediately to discuss the situation.

-- _____

_____

_____

-- _____

_____

_____

-- _____

_____

_____

Alternative Strategies for Jerry Silverman

--Send a memo to Betty Miles outlining your position, with no copies to anyone.

--Send a memo to Betty Miles outlining your position, with copies to the following persons:

_____	_____
_____	_____
_____	_____

--Call the Division Director above Betty Miles and ask for an immediate appointment with her.

--Call the Division Director above Betty Miles and ask her to write a memo to Betty Miles.

--Send a memo to the Division Director, with no copies to anyone.

--Send a memo to the Division Director, with copies to the following persons:

_____	_____
_____	_____
_____	_____

--Call the Division Director and ask her if she will go with you to see Betty Miles.

--Call Betty Miles and ask her to come and see you immediately.

-- _____

_____

_____

-- _____

_____

_____

-- _____

_____

_____

Step 2. Developing a Main Strategy (10 minutes)

The ego and alter-ego of Betty Miles should now meet to compare their chosen alternative strategies and to discuss their choices. Then the two of you together will develop a main strategy, either by choosing one or other of the alternative strategies or by combining strategies. The ego player has the final say.

The ego and alter-ego of Jerry Silverman should now do the same thing, compare their chosen alternatives, and develop a main strategy. Again, the ego player has the final say.

The organizational consultants should divide up in order to observe each pair of players and take notes, noting which aspects of the strategy are debilitative and which are productive. Do not participate in the ego/alter-ego discussion.

When the ego and alter-ego of both Betty Miles and Jerry Silverman have finished conferencing, write the main strategy in the space below.

For organizational consultants, write your notes in the space below.

_____

_____

_____

_____

_____

_____

_____

_____

_____

_____

When all of you have finished, proceed to Step 3.

Step 3. Reporting Main Strategies (10 minutes)

The ego players for Betty Miles and for Jerry Silverman will now reveal to each other the main strategy which they have developed. Be sure to include what you see as the possible consequences of your decision and why you chose what you did. First, Betty should share her position. Then Jerry should share his position. Then Betty has one response and Jerry has the final rebuttal. Remember, this exchange should only take 5 minutes.

Now the organizational consultants should give their report. Tell which aspects of the main strategies you think are debilitating and which are productive. If the strategies of the consultants are different from those presented by Betty Miles and Jerry Silverman, share them with the group. Include what the possible consequences of those strategies are and why you chose what you did.

When each of you has reported, move on to Step 4.

Step 4. Analysis of Strategies and Debriefing (10 minutes)

Recall all the alternatives Betty Miles had at her disposal. It is possible to delineate the relative merits of each alternative. Listed below are some of the most common alternatives available to any supervisor in a situation similar to Betty Miles's. After reading each of the strategies listed below, rank order them on your own without consulting other members of your group. If your group developed a strategy that does not appear in the list below, write your strategy below and include it in your ranking.

_____ a. A telephone call requesting an early appointment to discuss the situation.

_____ b. Immediate discussion in the subordinate's office.

_____ c. Immediate discussion in the supervisor's office.

_____ d. A memo from the supervisor to the subordinate reminding the subordinate of his/her obligation.

_____ e. Send the same memo as listed in "d" above, with a copy to a higher echelon.

_____ f. Alternative strategy _____

_____

_____

After each of you has rank-ordered these alternatives, turn to the next page.

Working as a group, discuss the answers to the following questions:

1. Compare your rankings of the alternatives with those found below. What is your reaction to this ranking? Do those of you who played the roles of Jerry Silverman and the consultants have different perspectives?

2. How does the use of threats affect organizational conflicts from the perspective of the subordinate as well as those at the higher echelons?

RANKING OF ALTERNATIVES

(Most preferred)

__1__	a.	A telephone call requesting an early appointment to discuss the situation is a preferred choice. Face to face discussion in an atmosphere of calm, unhurried objectivity is likely to bring the best results.
__2__	b.	Immediate discussion in the subordinate's office may catch him/her at a bad moment. On the other hand, he/she is in familiar surroundings with access to papers or other materials that he/she may wish to show you. Although there is some risk that lack of preparation may lead him/her to make some poorly considered responses, this approach should create an opportunity for discussing the problem constructively.
__3__	c.	Asking for an immediate discussion in your office has the same disadvantages as going to the subordinate's. Moreover, it brings the subordinate into a more threatening environment and, therefore, is even less desirable.
__4__	d.	A memo reminding the subordinate of his/her obligation is a somewhat impersonal step and may create resentment. It may bring some grudging, limited progress, but it does have the advantage of putting the supervisor's stance on paper and also gives the subordinate the same opportunity. This can be an advantage if it will be important later on to prove the position one says one has taken.
__5__ (Least preferred)	e.	Sending a copy of a memo to a higher echelon in order to increase its impact considerably worsens its effects upon the subordinate. In a situation such as the one portrayed in this frame, where the "opening rounds" of the conflict are taking place, it can be a poor choice indeed. In the "later rounds" of a conflict, it can serve as a fairly powerful level if force is needed with the subordinate.
_____	f.	Alternative Strategy _____

FRAME III

HANDLING INTERPERSONAL CONFLICT

Step 1. Analyzing a Subordinate's Reaction (15 minutes)

Working with your group of six, make sure that you are all situated as far away as possible from other groups so that you won't disturb each other.

Interpersonal conflict reveals itself most in face-to-face interaction. Both supervisors and subordinates can be the instigators of this conflict. A supervisor can approach subordinates generally in one of two ways:

- --open, supportive (sympathetic, attempting to draw out subordinate, empathetic);
- --closed, authoritarian (hostile, giving orders without allowing feedback, using one's position as reason why subordinate should obey).

A subordinate can respond in one of five ways. The subordinate can be:

- --ready to cooperate (actively offering to participate in the search for a solution to the problem);
- --defensive (justifying or explaining past behavior);
- --inclined to withdraw (avoiding the problem);
- --evasive (circumventing, eluding by dexterity or strategem);
- --hostile (accusing or angry tone; sullen).

It is possible that a situation could contain more than one type of reaction. For the purpose of this simulation, however, you will be working with only one type at a time.

Within your group, choose one person to be Person A and one person to be Person B to read a scripted dialogue. Person A will be the supervisor and will read out loud and slowly one statement at a time in order to allow for the response. Person B will be the subordinate and will respond with the response that is next to the statement made by Person A. Only Persons A and B should turn to the "Supervisor-Subordinate Dialogue."

The rest of the participants in the group will be evaluators and should mark on the "Evaluator's Guide" following the Dialogue according to (a) whether the supervisor's opening statement was open and supportive or closed and authoritarian and (b) whether the subordinate's statement was displaying a willingness to cooperate, defensiveness, an inclination to withdraw, evasiveness, or hostility.

When all the statements have been read and all members of the group have marked their choices, continue with this step.

SUPERVISOR-SUBORDINATE DIALOGUE

SUPERVISOR'S OPENING STATEMENT	SUBORDINATE'S REACTION
(Person A)	(Person B)

1. I am sympathetic to the fact that you are presented with a difficult situation. Can we discuss the situation and somehow clarify the problem?

    I've been trying to do the job, as you know, but I just can't seem to get together with the others that have responsibility in this matter. Which reminds me: have you talked to the other departments about their daily work schedules?

2. It seems to me that you've had plenty of time to solve this problem. When are you going to get it done?

    I wish you'd give this task to someone else. It's not my job to handle this situation.

3. Can you bring me up to date on the problems that you are encountering in this situation?

    You know I've been trying to take care of this, but it seems that I just can't get a handle on it. I need help. Yes, I would like to talk with you about the whole thing.

4. It seems to me that you are having some difficulty with this situation. Would you care to discuss it now, or do you want to think about your position for a few more days?

    As you know, I've got a lot of work to do. And I'm doing the best I can. When I can get to it, I will.

5. I thought you understood that the portion of the job was to be done by yesterday. I even sent you a memo with a timetable, and you never responded in a fashion that would indicate you couldn't do it.

    Get off it. Why the big rush? We've gotten along for years this way. I don't see why it matters if it takes only six months or so to get this worked out. People are always rushing me around here. It is hard to get anything done.

EVALUATOR'S GUIDE

Statements	Supervisor's Opening Statement		Subordinate's Response				
	open, supportive	closed, authoritarian	ready to cooperate	defensive	inclined to withdraw	evasive	hostile
1							
2							
3							
4							
5							

Take a minute now and allow the supervisor and the subordinate to tell the group how it felt to give and to receive some of the statements that were just made. Which ones were easiest to make, and which ones were hardest? Which ones felt the best, which ones the worst?

Now compare the answers you marked to this chart.

Statement	Supervisor	Subordinate
1	open	evasive
2	closed	withdrawal
3	open	cooperative
4	open	defensive
5	closed	hostile

If you did not understand why some of the opening statements or responses were classified the way they were, take just a few moments to discuss those statements with your group members. When you have finished this step, proceed to the next step.

Step 2. Analyzing Nonproductive Responses (5 minutes)

When your group has finished Step 1, select one of the four nonproductive responses (evasiveness, defensiveness, hostility, or withdrawal) which your group would like to learn to handle. Check the step which the entire group will work on.

_____ Step 3. Dealing with Defensiveness
_____ Step 4. Dealing with Evasiveness
_____ Step 5. Dealing with Withdrawal
_____ Step 6. Dealing with Hostility

When your group has finished working with one step, go on to another step if you have time. You may proceed to work on the first step you have chosen.

Step 3. Dealing with Defensiveness (20 minutes)

Problem. You are the supervisor of the outpatient service program at the Sandy Beach Community Mental Health Center. You hope to establish longer hours of regular service, at least open some evenings. This, you feel, could be accomplished by extending the hours of present staff and hiring one new typist. Your present treatment staff includes 2½ social workers, a psychiatrist, a psychologist, and a part-time crisis counselor. The social workers have refused to extend their hours, saying that they're already overworked. As evidence, they present a report showing that they have been carrying a caseload average of 100 cases per month, whereas the psychologist has been averaging 75 cases per month.

Assume that when questioned, the psychologist's response was essentially a defensive one. Example: "As you know, I've got a lot of work to do. I have always had to take on the cases that no one else will handle." He goes on to say: "I don't know what else I could do in addition to what I've been doing. Nobody is helping me with these cases--I'm sure I can't handle any more cases."

This type of defensive reaction usually has some underlying cause. It may result from self-doubt on the part of the subordinate, lack of confidence in his ability, or a vague fear of some perceived threat. It is always possible that what he is saying is true and that he is really too busy and overworked. In all probability, this is not the case; if it were, he would have come to you some time ago to ask for help in solving the problem. It is, therefore, likely that the defensive reaction is a screen for anxiety.

During your interview with your subordinate, you need to diagnose the situation by encouraging him to talk and your response could be:

OPTIONS

A. I think you are saying that you have too many demands on your time. However, let's zero in on this particular problem. If other relevant problems are involved, let's try to solve those, too.

B. I think you're telling me that you're really overburdened. However, I have the feeling that this might not be the basic reason for the problem.

C. I'd be less than candid with you if I didn't tell you that I think you could get this problem solved if you really wanted to.

D. You know that I would not have asked for your help in solving this problem if I didn't have a lot of confidence in you. I'm sure you can put this together right, and I would like you to tell me how you think I can help.

E. Can you tell me more about those other problems that are standing in the way of this one? What are they?

Sub-step 1. Individual Determination (5 minutes)

Without discussion, decide which statement is the one most likely to elicit the information you want from your subordinate so that an effort can then be made to solve the real problem behind the conflict. Circle the letter of your answer.

Sub-step 2. Group Discussion (10 minutes)

When everyone has marked his/her choice, each team member should tell the group what his/her choice was and the reason he/she had for making it.

When each team member has presented his/her selection and the discussion is complete, the team should then unanimously select a group response which they feel is best. Enter the letter here _____ and turn to the next page.

Sub-step 3. Analysis (5 minutes)

Analyze your personal and group choices as indicated below.

OPTIONS

A. This is a desirable approach. You are carrying the message that you understand the subordinate's problem and that you want to help him/her, so long as he/she is willing to discuss it with you frankly.

B. You may be right that what the subordinate has said is not the only reason for the problem. In making this analysis, you are interpreting his/her comment. Stating your interpretation of his/her words so bluntly, however, may have the opposite effect from the one you are seeking. The subordinate may conclude that you are going to be arbitrary in your inferences; and, in any case, people do not as a rule like to be told that they have reasons, other than the one they give, for what they say or do.

C. To declare that you think the subordinate can move faster than he/she has is to pass judgment before you have heard his/her side of the story. He/she may resent this; certainly, it is not the best way to bring about an open exchange of views or create an atmosphere in which problem solving becomes easy.

D. Expressing your confidence in the subordinate and thereby showing your willingness to support him/her is a desirable way to begin. It should reduce his/her anxiety about the discussion to follow.

E. Asking to be told more about the problem the subordinate is encountering is a good way to help him/her start talking and thereby lose some of his/her inhibitions and fears.

The chart below gives you the relative merit and main theme of
each of these statements.

Merit	Statement	Main Theme
Greatest	D	Supportive
	A and E	Understanding (A) Probing (E)
	B	Interpretive
Least	C	Judgmental

No one statement reflects an absolute right or wrong way to act as
a manager. Rather, your choice of statement may indicate a need for
balance on your part. For example, if your choice was interpretive,
you reflect an analytic style that may need to be more balanced with an
interpersonal, supportive, or understanding style.

When your group has finished this step, go on to the next step you
have chosen. If this is your second of the two steps you have chosen,
proceed to Step 7.

Step 4. Dealing with Evasiveness (30 minutes)

Problem. You are Director of Vocational Rehabilitation Services. Over the past few months one of your key staff members, Jan Starnes, has consecutively missed three staff meetings. This has created quite a problem for other staff members and for you, as over these past few months you and your staff have been preparing for workshops to be conducted around the country. You have recently called Jan in to inquire about the reasons for her nonattendance. Her response was: "I've tried to attend the meetings, as you know, but other responsibilities have interfered. Have you talked to the other staff members about assuming their share of the workload so that I will have the time to attend staff meetings?"

An evasive response such as this occurs either because your staff member does not want to attend the meetings, or because of some as yet undisclosed problem. In order to get your subordinate talking you can use a response that is:

1. Factual (searching for facts only);
2. Interpretive (analyzing the other person's behavior);
3. Judgmental (assessing the other person's behavior);
4. Understanding (demonstrating intellectual and emotional knowledge of the other's viewpoint);
5. Supportive (expressing sympathy).

Some of these responses, of course, will put her in a more communicative mood than others. Nevertheless, under certain circumstances, only one of them may be a good way to respond to her statement. A great deal depends on the relationship between you and her.

Sub-step 1. Individual Determination (5 minutes)

Without discussion, select two of the five response types listed above; then, utilizing these response approaches, write a few sentences indicating how you would respond after first indicating the approach you are going to use.

Response 1 (type _____): _____

_____

_____

_____

_____

_____

Response 2 (type _____): _____

_____

_____

_____

_____

_____

Sub-step 2. Individual Presentation (10 minutes)

After each person in the group has had a chance to develop his/her responses, begin to share your thoughts with each other with regard to the responses you wrote and why you considered them to be appropriate.

Sub-step 3. Group Determination (15 minutes)

After each member of the group has had a chance to make a presentation, the group should discuss the qualities of the various statements and then decide which statements seem to be the most appropriate. List those statements below:

_____

_____

_____

_____

_____

_____

_____

_____

_____

_____

When your group has finished this step, go on to the next step you have chosen. If this is your second of the two steps you have chosen, proceed to Step 7.

Step 5. Dealing with Withdrawal (25 minutes)

Problem. You are team leader for the children's unit at Sandy Beach Community Mental Health Center. Under recent expansion two new staff members have been added to the children's unit. The newer staff members have been especially interested in developing program changes which have been enthusiastically accepted by the children's team with the exception of the senior social worker, Russell Lewis. When you asked him how he felt about the changes he replied: "I simply don't agree with the program changes. These are not the kinds of things I should be doing. I don't want to see any changes made in our program."

Such a statement of withdrawal by the subordinate may hide apprehension about his lack of competence or his anxiety arising from various other sources. It may also be a symptom of hostility. Any negative response can, to some degree, signal these two possibilities. It is important to find out what is causing the subordinate's resistance before you decide on a course of action. Listed on the next page is a sequence of four steps. Read them carefully.

Sub-step 1. Individual Determination (5 minutes)

Without discussion, check the step or steps that you feel should be taken. (Any number of steps may be chosen.)

	Personal Choice	Group Choice
a. **Explanation with promise of support** Attempt to create a climate of understanding by making statements that indicate your support. Once you have gained your subordinate's confidence, use questions to try to get at the real cause of his/her resistance.		
b. **Explanation plus an appeal** Restate the problem, emphasizing the importance it has for the organization, and request that the subordinate further clarify his/her position relative to it.		
c. **An effort at persuasion** Restate the overall situation. Outline the advantages of this particular change, both for the organization as a whole and for the subordinate's own department, and attempt to influence him/her to reconsider his/her position.		
d. **A direct order** Explain to the subordinate that you are sorry he/she feels that he/she is not qualified to handle the situation, but no one else can do it, and, therefore, he/she must go ahead. Ask him/her to let you know if he/she needs any additional resources, technical advice, or budgetary support.		

Sub-step 2. Group Discussion (15 minutes)

After all the individual choices have been made, go around the group and discuss each person's choices and his/her reasons for making them.

After all the choices have been discussed, decide as a group what choices the group now thinks should be made. (Any number may be chosen.)

Sub-step 3. Analysis (5 minutes)

Three broad principles can be used to evaluate the choices of steps you as an individual and the choices you as a group made. These three principles are:

- --An order should not be issued until efforts (at least one of each type) have been made to explore the reasons for resistance, to offer support, and to persuade.
- --Threats should not be used until an order has been given.
- --Appeals are generally not as useful as expressions of support or persuasion.

Applying these principles to all the possible combinations of steps helps to identify the "best" combination of choices. The combinations are listed in order from the greatest relative merit to the least relative merit as follows:

GREATEST   LEAST

a-c-b-d; a-c-d; a-d; a-b-c; c-d; a-c; b; a; none

When your group has finished this step, go on to the next step you have chosen. If this is your second of the two steps you have chosen, proceed to Step 7.

Step 6. Dealing with Hostility (35 minutes)

Problem. Assume that you are administrator of a human service agency. Recently you have requested that each of your supervisors undertake with their staffs a comprehensive work sampling survey in order to meet federal requirements and regulations. The key section of your memo to staff explaining the rationale for this new requirement is as follows: "Current cost allocation plans require that we spend a certain percentage of our time performing specified functions to receive reimbursement for federal monies; thus it is mandatory that we undertake a comprehensive work sampling study to justify our expenditures."

Sub-step 1. (15 minutes)

Your memo initiated an uproar among a number of the supervisors. On the next pages are found a series of in-basket items which are replies to your memo regarding the working sampling survey. Each participant, as administrator, should read all of the in-basket items. Use these guidelines for your response to each item.

1. Read all the in-basket items. Write your response to each item in the space below.

2. If your response to an in-basket item is a letter or memo, write the content of the message just as you would at your office.

3. If your response to an in-basket item is a telephone call or personal contact, write the name of the person you would contact and the essence of your reply.

When all members of your group have finished this individual work, proceed to Sub-step 2.

MEMORANDUM "A"

TO: Administrator, Human Service Agency

FROM: Harold Chapman, Supervisor of Central Unit

RE: Work Sampling Survey

As you know, our programs are currently suffering from excessive staff caseloads. My staff has patiently attempted to comply with the incessant amount of paperwork which adds an intolerable burden to our workload. Already overburdened, I see no way that I can ask my staff to comply with this request. Under the circumstances, I am outraged at this additional pressure.

RESPONSE

_____ _____

_____

_____

_____

_____

_____

_____

MEMORANDUM "B"

TO: Administrator, Human Service Agency

FROM: Jan Davis, Director of Social Services

RE: Work Sampling Survey

I find it difficult to believe that an additional request for paperwork has been initiated. My staff is currently engaged in extensive data compilation required by the State Division of Family Services and I simply will not request that our staff undertake this additional burden at this time. I cannot understand why money and time must be spent in this manner when our resources are already badly depleted.

RESPONSE

_____

_____

_____

_____

_____

_____

_____

MEMORANDUM "C"

TO: Administrator, Human Service Agency

FROM: Katherine Starnes, Director of Protective Services Unit

RE: Work Sampling Survey

A request for additional "compliance with regulations" strikes me as an intolerable burden. My staff of professionally trained workers has patiently attempted to handle the ever-increasing amount of paperwork which emanates from federal, state, county, and hospital "procedural tasks." Hired as professionals, when can we perform the services for which we are trained? I would like to request a meeting with you, myself, and my staff as soon as possible in order to clarify my position on this matter.

RESPONSE

_____

_____

_____

_____

_____

MEMORANDUM "D"

TO: Administrator, Human Service Agency

FROM: Myron Gaines, Supervisor of Income Maintenance

RE: Work Sampling Survey

We don't have time to do this paperwork. I'm short two people and have to spend <u>all</u> my time supervising the people I <u>do</u> have. How do you expect me to do this "survey" when you don't give me enough money to hire the people I need to get the work done that we <u>already</u> have to do? Anyway, the whole thing doesn't make any sense.

RESPONSE

_____

_____

_____

_____

_____

_____

_____

Sub-step 2. Sharing of Individual Responses (10 minutes)

Within your group, you should share the responses you wrote to the in-basket items. Be prepared to share your rationale for the choices made with other group members. The group members may ask clarifying or explanatory questions, but do not get into an argument about the relative merits of each response.

Sub-step 3. Group Determination of the "Best" Responses (10 minutes)

After all the responses have been read, group members should decide by consensus which response among those read seems most appropriate for each of the four in-basket items. Jot down a summary of each of these responses below.

After the group has determined which are the "best" responses, outline the group's rationale for each of its choices. Write that rationale under each response in the lines below.

MEMORANDUM "A"

_____
Response

_____

_____
    Rationale

MEMORANDUM "B"

_____
Response

_____

_____
    Rationale

MEMORANDUM "C"

_____
Response
_____

_____
Rationale

MEMORANDUM "D"

_____
Response
_____

_____
Rationale

When your group has finished this step, go on to the next step you have chosen. If this is your second step of the two steps you have chosen, proceed to Step 7.

Step 7. Debriefing (10 minutes)

Answer the following questions within your small group:

1. In working with one or more nonproductive responses (de.~nsiveness, evasiveness, withdrawal, or hostility), you developed some general principles in how to work with those types of responses. What are these principles? Write them on the lines below.

_____

_____

_____

_____

_____

2. Why is it important for a supervisor to be skilled in analyzing a subordinate's response?

3. Which is easier for you to deal with, organizational conflict or interpersonal conflict?

ANSWERS TO FRAME I, STEP 1

1 - Negative; 2 - Positive; 3 - Positive; 4 - Negative

RELATED READINGS

Coser, L. W. The functions of social conflict. Glencoe, Ill.: The Free Press, 1956.

Webber, R. A. Managing organizational conflict. In National project on education for management. Philadelphia: Wharton Entrepreneurial Center, 1975.

3

TEACHING STAFF

I. INTRODUCTION

In its broadest sense, staff development can be defined as any program which will produce more effective behavior of workers on the job. Teaching is one method through which staff development can be accomplished.

With this in mind, this simulation offers participants an opportunity to examine the practical aspects of teaching staff by introducing the principles of a therapeutic community into existing treatment environments found in both state hospitals and community mental health centers. The principles of a therapeutic community represent a relatively new approach to improving the quality of patient care. Simulation participants will have an opportunity to experiment with a range of staff development activities. Effective supervisors and managers must also be educators whether involved in educating their staff or educating the community.

Staff development is an ongoing process of educating staff in order to improve the operation of the agency and contribute to the professional growth of all staff. All supervisors and administrators engage in some form of staff education. The person involved in staff development should have some knowledge of the nature of the adult learner, the teaching process, and the training process.

Teaching adults is different from teaching youth. The most obvious difference is that, while youth are preparing for life, adults are involved in life. Accordingly, adults have a wealth of experience which they use as a yardstick to measure anything that is new to them.

Education is no longer the central focus of a typical adult's life; education is ancillary and hence often viewed as a means to an end and judged primarily by its usefulness for immediate application. The adult usually possesses some negative memories of his/her prior formal education. As a result, the adult learner does not respond well to traditional modes of learning.

Keeping these characteristics of the adult learner in mind one can formulate some principles for the teaching process used with adults. The spirit in which learning takes place should be egalitarian, not authoritarian. The teacher should be a facilitator by drawing upon all participants in the search for knowledge; the knowledge of the teacher and the participants should be shared. Therefore, adults should be active participants in the learning process. Although a lecture is the best way to convey large amounts of information in a short period of time, techniques such as small group discussions and laboratory exercises are much more suited to the adult learner. Any information that is to be learned must be relevant to the work situation of the participant. Ideally, the information should be structured so that it builds upon skills and knowledge already possessed by the adult.

While working with people within their work setting is the most difficult way to bring about change, it appears to have the greatest impact on people. The change accomplished through in-service training experiences is most likely to be permanent. Removing individuals from their work setting (i.e., to a workshop) offers them a chance to experiment fairly safely, with the result that individual change will be brought about fairly quickly. Yet this change may more easily disappear when the individual resumes his role in the work setting. A staff developer, therefore, chooses wisely how and where he/she will attempt to bring about change by taking into account all the factors in the agency environment.

II. GOAL AND ENABLING OBJECTIVES

Goal:

To learn some of the principles and practices involved in teaching staff new approaches to service delivery.

Enabling Objectives:

1. Participants will demonstrate ability to teach key concepts of developing a therapeutic community to a trainee/learner.

2. Participants will demonstrate understanding of staff resistance to change and develop methods of meeting such resistance.

3. Participants will demonstrate knowledge of differing teaching strategies and demonstrate ability to apply this knowledge.

III. PROCEDURES

FRAME I - Preparing to Teach

Step 1. Background Information on the Therapeutic Community (10 minutes)
Step 2. Individual Task Preparation (15 minutes)
Step 3. Group Determination of Task (15 minutes)
Step 4. Debriefing (15 minutes)

FRAME II - Understanding Teaching Strategies

Step 1. Preparation for Developing a Teaching Strategy (10 minutes)
Step 2. Group Evaluation of Methods (15 minutes)
Step 3. First Training Session (30 minutes)

FRAME III - Staff Resistance to Change

Step 1. Individual Ranking of Resistance to Change (10 minutes)
Step 2. Reassessment through Group Discussion (15 minutes)
Step 3. Principles to Overcome Resistance: Individual Work (10 minutes)
Step 4. Principles to Overcome Resistance: Group Work (30 minutes)

FRAME IV - Debriefing (20 minutes)

FRAME I

PREPARING TO TEACH

In this frame, comprehension skills are called upon as participants work individually to understand the concepts involved in a therapeutic community and then, in groups, to strengthen their understanding through discussion.

Step 1. Background Information on the Therapeutic Community
     (Jones, 1968; Ellsworth, 1968) (10 minutes)

Staff development in an institution or organization has few beneficial results unless tied to a specific goal . . . in this case, the goal is the therapeutic community. Briefly defined, the therapeutic community is an ever-evolving environment wherein staff and clients meet in an open communication and decision-making process about the life of the community they share.

In the therapeutic community, staff and patients are afforded an unusual opportunity for discussion of behavior in treatment, administrative, and work settings. An unusual amount of time is set aside for the examination of the social structure of the community. In the therapeutic community, the role of the patient and each staff member is constantly under scrutiny, as are the role relationships among the various departments, disciplines, and subgroups in the community. New relationships are possible in many of the group meetings that can be established within the hospital or organization. Thus, in a review of a ward or therapeutic group meeting, there is an opportunity for learning and training through a discussion of role relationships of doctors, nurses, social workers, activity therapists, and patients. Furthermore, many of the staff are sensitized to the role of others which further increases the capacity to express feelings with a view to increase the effectiveness of patient care.

A therapeutic community, therefore, is one of continual learning--about oneself, about clients, about new techniques, programs, procedures, about each other--and it is the task of the professional to promote a therapeutic atmosphere open to the learning process.

One of the suggested ways to establish an open environment is the formation of in-house groups such as administrative, treatment, training, and work groups which meet frequently at appointed times and involve each segment of the community in communication and training. Apart from specific functions appropriate to each group, they operate on a basis of a two-way communication with the expression of feeling and an opportunity to discuss what is happening in the interactional situation freely. This discussion of a person's performance and feelings is not easy to attain since it goes against many cultural norms and it can often take a year or more for the ordinary staff member to talk about feelings and role performance with a view toward helping each other. This is a form of "positive criticism," but there is also a great deal of learning inherent in group communication processes for both patient and staff. There is learning about each other, learning to observe oneself, learning what prevents or provokes reactions in others, learning the responsibility each group member has to the group and to the group's function.

These various meetings of groups are linked by the overlapping of staff and patients in two or more groups. In this way, two-way communication is achieved from the level of the most regressed patient to the chief of the inpatient service.

Another way to maintain openness is to create decision-making machinery which allows for decentralization of many of the less important decisions to units where problems exist or to group meetings where all voices are heard and all feelings aired prior to taking action. It is important to understand that the ultimate decision-making machinery regarding major problems rests with senior staff groups. These upper level decisions are based on needs as expressed at lower levels that have been reported up the line. It should also be remembered that oftentimes administrative decisions and therapy overlap and decision-making machinery must reflect these two functions. For instance, decisions such as the suitability of a patient's weekend pass or the transfer of a psychiatric aide are an integral part of therapy and they call for a high degree of integration between patients and staff. This kind of decision involves both segments of the community and both should be heard.

Other decisions involve only staff, but here also there is need for openness in allowing for inclusion of judgments and opinions of all staff, including janitorial and maintenance personnel, to play a part in determining final action. In this way, all staff begin to feel the importance of team effort because they are truly a part of the team. Continued effort in this direction will break down the traditional bureaucratic atmosphere of institutions and organizations that handle many patients and will erase the need for the defensive attitudes on the part of staff who have felt isolated from the policy level and have created barriers to protect themselves on the job from decisions that come down from the top.

A good communication system that is coupled with a democratic decision-making policy thereby becomes the underpinnings of a therapeutic community where everyone is involved in a more active and responsible role. In this way, life within an institution or organization.becomes a living laboratory where crises, instead of being seen as troublesome, can be turned into learning situations and opportunities to meet training needs. And in turn the learning and training further increases the evolutionary process of communicating and deciding in a day-to-day fashion in order to maintain an atmosphere of learning and rehabilitation.

Basic to the concept of the therapeutic community is the idea of involving all persons, including patients and staff, in the planning and implementation of treatment programming.

Step 2. Individual Task Preparation (15 minutes)

As individuals, without discussion, you are to assume the role of a staff trainer. You have just finished presenting and discussing the above material in a staff meeting on the children's ward. In order to insure that staff members have understood the material, you will prepare five (5) questions of a somewhat specific nature as a quick quiz. This exercise requires not only that you understand the material but also that you be able to organize the material into its pertinent concepts so that the questions cover what you think is the important material for staff to retain. Be sure to include questions that cover both knowledge of the content and application of the content.

1. _____

_____

2. _____

_____

3. _____

_____

4. _____

_____

5. _____

_____

Step 3. Group Determination of Task (15 minutes)

All participants should divide into two or three small groups.
As a group, determine through discussion what five questions should be
included in the quiz to insure that the material has been covered and
that the staff will be able to apply the material.

1. _____

_____

2. _____

_____

3. _____

_____

4. _____

_____

5. _____

_____

After all groups have chosen their list of five questions, have
one spokesperson from each group read its questions aloud to the
combined groups.

<u>Step 4. Debriefing</u> (15 minutes)

Staying within your group, answer the following questions:

1. Review the questions you formulated by yourself in Step 2 and as a group in Step 3.

		Individual	Group
A.	How many questions began with "who"?	_____	_____
B.	How many questions began with "what"?	_____	_____
C.	How many questions began with "why"?	_____	_____
D.	How many questions began with "how"?	_____	_____
E.	Were the questions generally concrete or abstract?	_____	_____
F.	Were the questions usually specific or general?	_____	_____

2. As you worked in your group, what kind of decision-making process did you use to choose the five questions? Did you vote, or acquiesce, or what?

FRAME II

UNDERSTANDING TEACHING STRATEGIES

In the last frame, participants analyzed the concepts of a
therapeutic community and discussed different approaches to assessing
staff's understanding of these concepts. This frame seeks to increase
one's understanding of teaching strategies. Teaching staff is an
integral part of administration and a major tool used in seeking to
implement change. In this frame, participants will explore the use of
different teaching strategies.

Step 1. Preparation for Developing a Teaching Strategy (10 minutes)

Participants should divide into teams of two (2) to prepare
teaching plans to meet the following situation. Each of you are
trainers on inpatient wards and must present the basic concepts of a
therapeutic community to the staff. In order to begin planning for
your first three training sessions, you need to assess a range of
instructional methods. There are two equally important considerations
you must keep in mind: imparting the content of the presentation and
overcoming resistance.

From the following list of teaching strategies, choose the
strategies you would use to introduce the new concepts of total staff
and patient involvement in a therapeutic community for the first three
training sessions. You may add to your list of strategies if you like.
Write the numbers of the strategies next to each training session.

1. Trainees illustrate concepts in art form

2. A 10-minute factual presentation

3. Examples drawn from personal experiences with staff

4. Trainees asked to paraphrase material presented in written form

5. Outline of ideas on chalk board

6. Role playing by instructor

7. Trainees engage in memory drill

8. Trainee summarizes procedures for the group

9. Trainees and instructor join in conversation circle

10. Trainees play a simulation game

11. Instructor lectures

12. Instructor draws conclusion and summarizes

13. Instructor calls for questions

14. Trainees ask for additional insight

    (other strategies--indicate what they are)

15. _____

16. _____

17. _____

Training Session #1 _____
                              strategy (ies)

Training Session #2 _____
                              strategy (ies)

Training Session #3 _____
                              strategy (ies)

<u>Step 2. Group Evaluation of Methods</u> (15 minutes)

You and your partner should now regroup into groups of six in order to compare notes on the teaching strategies selected for each training session. Based on this discussion, seek consensus on the three most appropriate strategies for each training session.

Training Session #1 _____

_____

_____

Training Session #2 _____

_____

_____

Training Session #3 _____

_____

_____

Step 3. First Training Session (30 minutes)

This step involves role playing the first training session. Each person in your group should assume one of these roles:

1. Staff trainer;
2. Supervisory ward nurse;
3. Ward psychiatrist;
4. Ward social worker;
5. Senior ward psychiatric technician;
6. Student intern.

Turn to the appropriate page for your role description and review it. To begin the role play, move around the circle and have each participant identify his/her role and the perspective(s) inherent in that role. After this is completed, the staff trainer should identify which teaching strategies were agreed upon in the previous step for this first training session and then briefly outline the main concepts behind a therapeutic community. When the ward trainer has completed his/her presentation, the floor will be open for questions and discussion. Some persons will be afraid of how the therapeutic community will change their jobs. Others will resent their seeming loss of power. Some persons will be ready to adopt the idea immediately. Others will favor the idea but will want to be cautious about its implementation.

1. Staff Trainer

You have developed and held many other training sessions, but this is your first experience with a therapeutic community. You are enthusiastic about the idea and think it would be a great thing for inpatient wards to use. As your academic career was spent in education, you have had limited direct contact with patients and experience in one-to-one treatment situations. You know that the director of the mental health agency which is responsible for this ward strongly favors the therapeutic community approach.

The main concepts of a therapeutic community are:

1. Open communication;
2. Open decision-making process;
3. Continual learning;
4. Sharing of power;
5. Involvement of both staff and patients.

2. Supervisory Ward Nurse

As the person responsible for the majority of the staff on the ward, you think you are interested in the therapeutic community concept but are quite apprehensive about changing the ward routine. You have experienced considerable turnover in the nursing ranks and fear that new therapeutic ideas will increase the flight of nursing personnel from the ward. You also wonder about how the therapeutic community will change the relationship between nurses and patients.

3. Ward Psychiatrist

Your time spent on the ward, since you are available only for rounds each morning, reflects interest primarily in the medication levels of the patients. Yet your position carries much status. All the staff continuously turn to you for both verbal and nonverbal approval of anything which relates to treatment. You learned about the therapeutic community approach during your residency and would like to support the development of this approach on the ward.

4. Ward Social Worker

As the ward social worker, you maintain an office on the ward and involve patients in individual therapy sessions and frequently involve family members. Occasionally, you conduct psychodrama sessions in the day room on the ward. You and the ward psychiatrist rarely see each other, much less confer. You feel that you do the majority of therapy on the ward. Your interest is primarily individual psychotherapy, but you might be interested in the new therapeutic community idea.

5. Senior Ward Psychiatric Technician

As the senior psychiatric technician, you have spent many years working with disturbed patients. While your observations are valued by the nursing staff, you have never been involved in planning a treatment program for individual patients or groups of patients. You're not sure that the ward psychiatrist even knows your name. And you know that the staff trainer has not had any of the type of experience you have had in dealing with patients.

6. Student Intern

You have been interning on this ward for the last two weeks. You are eager to apply all the ideas you have read about in school, particularly that of the therapeutic community. Although you know you are somewhat new to the situation, you still have a penchant for asking embarrassing questions, like "why aren't there any patients involved in this meeting?"

FRAME III

STAFF RESISTANCE TO CHANGE

Staff development is a process of change. Whenever change is proposed, resistance is certain to arise. Resistance to change is a natural phenomenon. It is unrealistic for anyone who seeks to make changes to proceed on the assumption that everyone can see the logic behind the change and hence accept it.

A concept such as the therapeutic community is sure to arouse resistance, as the implementation of a therapeutic community means that staff will need to change some very basic ways of working and relating on the job.

Participants have learned that communication and decision making are key elements that make up the structure of a therapeutic community. Open communication and a democratic form of decision making lend themselves to the creation of an environment wherein both staff and patients are continually learning together to solve problems in a way that meets the therapeutic needs of all. In this frame, participants will assume the role of the Chief of the Inpatient Service and will experience the resistance to change that introduction of daily, 8:00 a.m. senior staff meetings create among the staff.

Step 1. Individual Ranking of Resistance to Change (10 minutes)

As Chief of Inpatient Service, you have initiated daily, half-hour meetings with senior staff to establish communication links with all program areas and to get an overview of the problems and projects scheduled for that day. This process has been operating for three weeks and you have found the following problems. Rank each of these problems in the left-hand column from 1 to 6, with 1 indicating the most disruptive to the staff meeting, and 6 indicating the least disruptive to the staff meeting.

A. _____   Three staff members have complained that the Conference Room is inadequately heated in the morning and want afternoon meetings.   _____ A.

B. _____   The director of Nursing Services and the supervising physician have carried their schism into the open to the embarrassment of other staff members.   _____ B.

C. _____   The Occupational Therapy director has made it known, outside the meeting, that staff meetings every day are a waste of time that could be better used in treating patients.   _____ C.

D. _____   Absenteeism began to increase in the second week of meetings.   _____ D.

E. _____   Complaints have been registered, in the meetings, that staff sessions resemble sensitivity groups and this shows a lack of confidence on the part of the Chief in the abilities of senior staff to deal openly with peer group members.   _____ E.

F. _____   One department supervisor states there will be no decentralization of decision making in her area since junior staff lack the training and experience to make reliable judgments about patient treatment or administrative procedures.   _____ F.

Step 2. Reassessment through Group Discussion (15 minutes)

Rejoin your small group and share your ranking with others without discussion. This simulates the decision-making process where opinions of others, particularly staff, have been sought and received. Reassess your ranking in light of alternative opinions and return to the previous page and note them in the right-hand column.

Can you identify any of the problem areas as functional or useful in facilitating improved communications over time?

Step 3. Principles to Overcome Resistance to Change: Individual Work (10 minutes)

Assume that you are a consultant who has been asked by the Chief of Inpatient Service to work on the following problem:

> In an effort to institute a therapeutic community, the Chief of Inpatient Service has tried to initiate daily, half-hour meetings with senior staff (director of Nursing, Occupational Therapy director, chief psychiatrist, chief social worker, etc.). The meetings have been conducted for three weeks, with absenteeism continuing to increase with each succeeding meeting. Those who attend the meetings complain that they resemble sensitivity groups.

Each member in your group should choose two (2) numbers between 1 and 9. Members can choose the same numbers, but be certain that each number between 1 and 9 has been chosen.

After all members of the group have chosen two numbers, begin work individually. You will work together as a group in the next step; for now, work by yourself.

Turn to the "Principles for Change" on the following pages. According to the numbers you have chosen, you should:

1. read the principle;

2. apply this principle to the situation described above and write down your application. How would you operationalize this principle in the situation given?

When each member of your group has completed his/her work on each of his/her two principles, move on to the next step.

Principles for Change

(Fairweather, Sanders, & Tornatzky, 1974)

1. Try to get a number of people including those who have informal leadership involved in discussion and consideration of the innovation. Maximize participation and then gradually focus toward concrete action.

2. Be skeptical of verbal promises on the part of others regarding the acceptance of change. Verbal change is not the same as real change from old institutional roles to new ones.

3. Make your initial attempts at change in the organization in a limited way both in intensity and scope, and then gradually increase the action and commitment required.

4. Don't worry excessively about seducing the powers-that-be in the organization. You may, or may not, need their support, but don't focus exclusively on them.

5. Work to develop a support group, or focus attention on a pre-existing group that could become the support group. Concentrate on their viability as a group.

6. In replicating a training program from another agency or from another part of the country, feel free to borrow and adapt despite the fact that your agency may be quite different from the one in which the original training program was developed.

7. Your change activities will probably arouse the anxieties of some persons within the organization. Try to alleviate this condition.

8. You should try to ameliorate undue anxieties, but do not yield to pressure to modify the major dimensions of a therapeutic community so that the end product will be so watered down it will not work well.

9. Develop a technique to "pick yourself up off the floor" quickly and effortlessly when knocked down. Perseverance may not pay off but change cannot occur without it.

Step 4. Principles to Overcome Resistance to Change: Group Work
        (30 minutes)

Now is the time for the individuals in your group to share their responses to the list of principles. Start with the first principle. Have one person in the group read the principle aloud. Then each person who worked on that principle should share his/her applications. Take about 3 minutes per principle.

FRAME IV

<u>DEBRIEFING</u>

Working as an entire group, take 20 minutes to answer the following questions:

1. What is your reaction to the role play in the second frame? How realistic were the roles? How realistic was the type and amount of resistance?

2. What do you think is the most important principle for overcoming resistance?

3. While you were working in groups, were you functioning as a therapeutic community? How well did your group adhere to the basic concepts of a therapeutic community?

REFERENCES

Jones, M. Beyond the therapeutic community. New Haven, Conn.: Yale University Press, 1968, pp. 1-22.

Ellsworth, R. B. Non-professionals in psychiatric rehabilitation. New York: Appleton-Century-Crofts, 1968, pp. 43-60.

Fairweather, G. W., Sanders, D. H., & Tornatzky, L. A. Creating change in mental health organizations. New York: Pergamon Press, 1974, pp. 194-195.

RELATED READINGS

Brieland, D., Briggs, T., & Leuenberger, P. The team model of social work practice, Monograph no. 5. Syracuse, N. Y.: Syracuse University School of Social Work, 1973.

Brill, N. I. Working with people: The helping process. Philadelphia: J. P. Lippincott, 1973.

Caplan, G. An approach to community mental health. New York: Grune & Stratton, Inc., 1961.

Jones, M. Maturation of the therapeutic community: An organic approach to health and mental health. New York: Human Sciences Press, 1976.

Joyce, B., & Weil, M. Models of teaching. Englewood Cliffs, N. J.: Prentice-Hall, 1972.

Knowles, M. The modern practice of adult education. New York: Association Press, 1971.

Lassey, W. R. (Ed.). Leadership and social change. Iowa City, Iowa: University Associates Press, 1971.

Lynton, R. P., & Pareek, U. Training for development. Homewood, Ill.: The Dorsey Press, 1967.

Mager, R. F. Preparing objectives for programmed instruction. San Francisco: Fearon Publishers, 1972.

Magner, G. W., & Briggs, T. L. (Eds.). Service development in mental health services. New York: National Association of Social Workers, 1966.

Purvine, M. (Ed.). Educating MSW students to work with other social welfare personnel. New York: Council on Social Work Education, 1973.

Riessman, F., Cohen, J., & Pearl, A. Mental health of the poor. New York: The Free Press, 1964.

4

FINANCIAL ANALYSIS

I. PURPOSE

This simulation provides an opportunity to work on some of the
same problems which confront administrators of community mental health
programs and state mental hospital programs. The experience of dealing
with some realistic financial management problems in this simulation
should prove to be valuable in coping with similar situations in real
life. This simulation will provide participants with some experiences
that are relevant to those found in the management of either a
comprehensive community mental health center or a state mental
hospital. The administrator of either one of these organizations uses
skills in developing and managing a budget for program effectiveness as
well as managing multiple funding sources including federal, state,
local, voluntary, insurance, and fees.

II. GOAL AND ENABLING OBJECTIVES

Goal:

To acquaint participants with line-item and program budgeting and to give them experience in working with each type of budget.

Enabling Objectives:

1. To understand line-item and program budgets

2. To be able to analyze line-item budgets and convert them to program budgets

3. To gain experience in contingency planning

4. To learn to cost out programs

III. PROCEDURES

FRAME I - Types of Budgeting

Step 1. Understanding the Differences (10 minutes)
Step 2. Group Role Play (10 minutes)

FRAME II - Budget Analysis

Step 1. Individual Analysis (15 minutes)
Step 2. Staff Meeting (15 minutes)
Step 3. Program Budgeting (30 minutes)

FRAME III - Contingency Planning

Step 1. Individual Planning (5 minutes)
Step 2. Group Sharing (25 minutes)

FRAME IV - Costing Out Services

Step 1. Budget Calculations (10 minutes)
Step 2. Program Budget Preparation (20 minutes)
Step 3. Budget Alternatives (20 minutes)

FRAME V - Debriefing (20 minutes)

FRAME I

TYPES OF BUDGETING

Introduction

You have just been hired as a budget analyst in the Bureau of Financial Management in the State Division of Mental Health which is located in a large state human service agency. You've never had this kind of job before and so you are a little nervous. After one day at your new job, you rush home and frantically telephone an old friend of yours from school who knew a lot about budgeting. She has sent you a brief summary of line-item and program budgeting and even included a sample of each. You sneak these papers, which appear on the next few pages, into the office, as you know you'll need to refer to them from time to time.

Step 1. Understanding the Differences (10 minutes)

Read the exhibit which follows these questions. Then, individually, write down the answers to the following questions:

1. Which type of budgeting, line-item or program, allows for greater control over exactly how each dollar is spent?

   _____

2. Which type of budgeting can be blended more smoothly into the planning process?

   _____

3. What are the classifications used in line-item budgeting?

   _____in program budgeting?_____

4. Which type of budgeting forces you to ask the question, "As an agency, what are we doing and how well are we doing it?"

   _____

Types of Budgets

The most common types of budgets in use today are line-item and program. You'll probably come across both types while you are a budget analyst. In some states more than one type is used. For example, in some states all budget requests from the agencies and budget recommendations from the Governor are program budgets, but the Legislature's appropriations bill is line-item.

Line Item

Line-item budgeting focuses on the "things" on which money is spent--personnel, operating expenses, fixed capital outlay, etc. It doesn't really tell you what an agency does; it just tells you how an agency spends its money. Most line-item budgets are incremental budgets, which means that the analysts concentrate on deciding what percentage increase each line should get for the next budget year. Line-item budgets assume that: (1) what the agency is doing is proper and worthwhile; and (2) that the efficiency or effectiveness of the agency can be measured primarily through the budgeting process.

In these times of diminishing resources and increasing demands, however, line-item budgeting (which has been used for many, many years) is coming under increasing fire. More and more agency officials are coming to view dollars spent as statements of value, and line-item budgets do not allow officials to make these types of value judgments. For example, saying that the Division of Mental Health spends $1,500 a year on maintenance of typewriters does not necessarily indicate the priorities of the agency.

In addition, line-item budgeting does not allow officials to examine alternatives to reaching an agency's goal. Listing the total amount spent on duplicating and xeroxing does not give you any idea how other service components in the budget are viewed (e.g., contracting out for psychological testing compared to conducting all psychological testing in-house).

In summary, then, line-item budgeting indicates the categories of expenditures but does not indicate the priorities of the agency, how well the agency is doing its job, or what alternatives (and the consequences of those alternatives) are available to the agency.

Program (or PPBS)

PPBS stands for Planning-Programming Budgeting Systems. It originated in the Department of Defense and has since spread to many states. As its name implies, planning of programs is the primary focus. Decisions about program objectives and the range of alternatives are identified before the budget is even begun. In one sense, then, the actual budget is a routine exercise that is the very last step in planning.

The program budget reflects a different format from the line-item budget. It covers several years, rather than just one. It tells you what the main goal of the agency is and it gives you performance effectiveness measures so you can tell how well the agency is doing its job. The dollar amounts are listed under the programs of the agency (such as rehabilitation of youthful offenders), not under the categories of expenditure (such as long distance telephone calls). It also gives a cost estimate for future years of the program, as well as future estimated effectiveness measures.

You can make the following type of statement with a program budget that simply cannot be made with a line-item budget: "We are presently rehabilitating 40% of our youthful offenders at $3,000 per youth per year, for a total yearly cost of $150,000. 'Rehabilitated' is defined as not having contact with the courts within five years after release from the program. We estimate that the number of youthful offenders will increase 8% per year. Taking into account an inflation factor of 10% per year, we can continue to rehabilitate 40% of our youthful offenders next year at a cost of $177,000. We can rehabilitate 50% of our youthful offenders at a cost of $200,000." In a line-item budget, a program such as rehabilitation of youthful offenders would be split into categories of expenditure (such as salaries, expenses, and capital outlay) and then lumped with other programs' categories of expenditure.

To identify specific funds spent on rehabilitation of youthful offenders is almost impossible in a line-item budget. And even if you did identify the amount of money out of the line-item budget, you would still have no idea how successfully the agency achieved its goals.

The following chart may help you understand the differences between line-item and program budgeting better.

APPROACH TO BUDGETING (Howard, 1973)

	Type of Budget Document	
	Line-Item	Program
Aspect of budget cycle stressed	Execution	Decisions before preparation
Budget classifications used	Line-item or object	Program
Skills stressed in budgeting	Accounting	Economics and system analysis
Time period covered	Usually one year	Multi-year
Characteristics of budget process	Control	Planning

EXAMPLE OF LINE-ITEM BUDGET

Department of Health and Rehabilitative Services
Division of Mental Health
General Office and Community Mental Health Program

Line Item	Estimated 1977-78	Requested 1978-79
Salaries and Benefits:	$	$
General Revenue Fund	2,139,672	2,732,592
Federal Aid Trust Fund	304,579	
Grants & Donations Trust Fund	273,714	396,338
Total Salaries and Benefits	2,717,965	3,128,930
Other Personal Services:		
General Revenue Fund	372,207	566,073
Grants & Donations Trust Fund	4,431	212,431
Total Other Personal Services	376,638	778,504
Expenses:		
General Revenue Fund	985,364	1,607,265
Federal Aid Trust Fund	2	
Grants & Donations Trust Fund	440,877	107,313
Total Expenses	1,426,243	1,714,578
Data Processing Services:		
General Revenue Fund	236,629	282,972
Operating Capital Outlay:		
General Revenue Fund	14,377	26,100
Grants & Donations Trust Fund	10,000	8,427
Total Operating Capital Outlay	24,377	34,527
Special Categories:		
Community Mental Health Services		
General Revenue Fund	9,290,372	18,435,922
Operations and Maintenance		
Trust Fund	3,040,600	2,050,000
Federal Aid Trust Fund	3,294,028	6,449,694
Grants & Donations Trust Fund		221,000
Total Community Mental Health Serv.	15,625,000	27,156,616
Community Alcoholic Services		
General Revenue Fund	3,368,320	9,327,610
Federal Aid Trust Fund	3,103,493	2,616,265
Grants & Donations Trust Fund	1,500,023	1,158,156
Total Community Alcoholic Serv.	7,971,836	13,102,031

Line Item	Estimated 1977-78	Requested 1978-79
	$	$
Purchased Client Services		
General Revenue Fund	2,767,752	2,737,196
Federal Aid Trust Fund	6,859,212	8,211,589
Total Purchased Client Services	9,626,964	10,948,785
Total By Funds:		
General Revenue Fund	19,174,693	35,715,730
Operation & Maintenance Trust Fund	3,040,600	2,050,000
Federal Aid Trust Fund	13,561,314	17,277,548
Grants & Donations Trust Fund	2,229,045	2,103,665
Total All Funds	$38,005,652	$57,146,943

EXAMPLE OF PROGRAM BUDGET

Department of Health and Rehabilitative Services
Division of Mental Health
General Office and Community Mental Health Program

Title of Program	Estimated 1977-78	Requested 1978-79
	$	$
Community Mental Health Services	26,518,851	39,831,900
Community Alcoholic Services	8,516,417	13,815,765
Public Education Services	173,049	177,414
Development of Mental Health Manpower	408,095	603,864
Dissemination of Knowledge in Mental Health	54,828	57,464
Administrative Direction and Support Services	2,334,412	2,660,536
Total All Program Components	$38,005,652	$57,146,943

Step 2. Group Role Play (10 minutes)

The answers to the four questions are as follows:

1. Line-Item - Every dollar is accounted for in every expense category.

2. Program - Its statement of goals and objectives and its measures of effectiveness match those of the planning process.

3. Line-Item Classifications - Line-item or objects such as personnel, rent, supplies, etc.

   Program Classifications - Program descriptions in terms of service goals and objectives.

4. Program - It speaks to what the agency is doing as a whole, not to how much money it's spending on pencils.

After reviewing your responses, divide into groups of four persons each. Within each group, assign two persons to Team A and two persons to Team B. Team A will be proponents of line-item budgeting and Team B will be proponents of program budgeting.

For the next 10 minutes, discuss among yourselves the advantages and disadvantages of line-item and program budgeting. Be sure to include different points of view in your discussion--that of legislative budget analysts, an agency budget analyst, a governor, an agency head. Each team should do its best to persuade the other team, but don't get into a violent argument. The purpose of this discussion is to get a good grasp on each type of budgeting by thoroughly exploring all advantages.

FRAME II

BUDGET ANALYSIS

As a budget analyst employed by the State Division of Mental Health, your job is to assist the division director with the management of mental health program funds. A request has recently been forwarded to you from the legislature in which several freshman legislators interested in mental health programs have asked for budget information. Specifically, they would like an explanation of the budgets currently used by community mental health centers and state mental hospitals.

Your boss, the Chief of the Bureau of Financial Management, has decided that this request is both urgent and instructive. Therefore, she has asked all her analysts to work on the response.

Step 1. Individual Analysis (15 minutes)

As you sit at your desk reviewing the budget materials in Exhibits 1 and 2 located at the end of this frame (one for a community mental health center and the other for a state hospital), develop an initial analysis. First, identify the service goals for each of these agencies, inferring these goals from the budgets which relate to the mental health service system. Next, list the similarities and differences between the two budgets. (Hint: One of the key similarities or differences can be line-item or program budgeting.)

SERVICE GOALS
(Mental Health Center)

1. _____

   _____

2. _____

   _____

3. _____

   _____

SERVICE GOALS
(State Hospital)

1. _____

_____

2. _____

_____

3. _____

_____

SIMILARITIES

1. _____

_____

2. _____

_____

3. _____

_____

DIFFERENCES

1. _____

_____

2. _____

_____

3. _____

_____

Step 2. Staff Meeting (15 minutes)

A staff meeting has been called to pool the best thinking for the purpose of developing a comprehensive response to the legislative request. Each participant should share his/her list of service goals, similarities, and differences. It is important to make notes on the ideas of others so that consensus can be reached after each participant has spoken.

SERVICE GOALS
(Mental Health Center)

1. _____
   _____
2. _____
   _____
3. _____
   _____

SERVICE GOALS
(State Hospital)

1. _____
   _____
2. _____
   _____
3. _____
   _____

SIMILARITIES

1. _____
   _____
2. _____
   _____
3. _____
   _____

DIFFERENCES

1. _____
   _____
2. _____
   _____
3. _____
   _____

Step 3. Program Budgeting (30 minutes)

In this step you should remain in the same groups as for Step 2 of this frame. For the first 15 minutes, assume that all of you work for the Tri-County Mental Health Center. The Chairman of the Board has called to ask that you make a presentation at the next board meeting in order to illustrate how the current budget of the Center could be described in program terms. For 15 minutes, work on her request. Write your sample budget format on the next page.

For the last 15 minutes of this step, assume that you all work in the financial management office in the Northern District State Hospital. The Superintendent has asked you to work up a sample budget format, showing how the hospital's current budget could be described in program terms. Work up a sample budget format on the page after next.

SAMPLE BUDGET FORMAT - COMMUNITY MENTAL HEALTH CENTER

PROGRAMS	COSTS	OUTPUT/BENEFITS

1.

2.

3.

4.

5.

SAMPLE BUDGET FORMAT - STATE HOSPITAL

PROGRAMS	COSTS	OUTPUT/BENEFITS
1.		
2.		
3.		
4.		
5.		

EXHIBIT 1   <u>COMPUTATION OF TOTAL BUDGET REQUEST</u>
<u>Fiscal Year Ending: June 30, 1976</u>

TRI-COUNTY COMMUNITY MENTAL HEALTH CENTER

Sources of Funding	Current Program Year Ending June 30, 1978	Requested Year Ending June 30, 1979
1. State funds requested	$172,801	$188,910
2. Local matching funds from tax-supported sources (counties and cities)	141,260	312,374
3. Estimated fees collected (not matchable)	121,549	105,881
4. Federal funds to be used in program (not matchable)	15,569	15,510
5. Other monies (DVR, sales, etc.) (not matchable)	0	0
6. Other contributions (associations, clubs, individuals, etc.)	17,974	12,569
7. TOTAL BUDGET	469,153	635,244

TRI-COUNTY COMMUNITY MENTAL HEALTH CENTER

Total Expenditures	Current Program Year Ending June 30, 1978	Requested Year Ending June 30, 1979
Administrative services	$ 67,440	$ 94,806
Mental health services	330,680	447,977
Aftercare services	28,162	28,622
Drug abuse program	42,871	63,839
TOTAL BUDGET	469,153	635,244

Computation of Program Operations for Administrative Services		
	Current Program Year Ending June 30, 1978	Requested Year Ending June 30, 1979
20 CONTRACTUAL SERVICE		
21 General Repair	180	72
22 Professional Service (Consultants)	0	0
23 Gas, Power, & Water (Public Utilities)	900	0
24 Traveling (Routine)	2,200	1,190
25 Traveling (Convention & Conference)	600	810
26 Communications (Tel. & Postage)	1,600	1,072
27 Printing--Other than office supplies	100	110
28 Other Contractual Services	700	4,030
TOTAL	$6,280	$7,284

30 SUPPLIES		
31 Fuel Supply	0	0
32 Office Supplies	1,000	1,500
33 Medical and Lab Supplies	0	0
34 Cleaning Supplies	50	130
35 Building Maintenance Supplies	0	0
36 Educational and Recreational Supplies	0	0
37 Other Supplies	0	0
TOTAL	1,050	1,630

40 EQUIPMENT		
41 Office Equipment	1,000	850
42 Medical & Laboratory Equipment	0	0
43 Educational & Recreational Equipment	0	0
44 Books and Periodicals	150	150
TOTAL	1,150	1,000

50 CHARGES AND OBLIGATIONS		
51 Rent	6,000	6,000
52 Insurance (Liability)	0	155
53 Dues, Memberships, & Subscriptions	125	135
54 Unclassified	0	0
TOTAL	6,125	6,290

PROFESSIONAL, PERSONNEL, AND OTHER EXPENDITURES		
10 Personnel Services (see attached)	$52,835	$78,602
20 Contractual Services	6,280	7,284
30 Supplies	1,050	1,630
40 Equipment	1,150	1,000
50 Charges and Obligations	6,125	6,290
TOTAL	$67,440	$94,806

Computation of Program Operations for Mental Health Services		
	Current Program Year Ending June 30, 1978	Requested Year Ending June 30, 1079
20 CONTRACTUAL SERVICE		
21 General Repair	663	300
22 Professional Service (Consultants) In-Patient*	15,000	30,000
23 Gas, Power, & Water (Public Utilities)	1,000	2,535
24 Traveling (Routine)	1,500	2,350
25 Traveling (Convention & Conference)	2,000	3,650
26 Communications (Tel. & Postage)	3,000	3,344
27 Printing-Other than office supplies	150	310
28 Other Contractual Services	1,015	9,903
TOTAL	$24,328	$52,392
30 SUPPLIES		
31 Fuel Supply	0	0
32 Office Supplies	1,300	1,000
33 Medical and Lab Supplies	1,145	300
34 Cleaning Supplies	150	450
35 Building Maintenance Supplies	0	300
36 Educational and Recreational Supplies	1,600	750
37 Other Supplies	0	400
TOTAL	4,195	3,200
40 EQUIPMENT		
41 Office Equipment	2,369	6,140
42 Medical & Laboratory Equipment	0	0
43 Educational & Recreational Equipment	2,450	1,100
44 Books and Periodicals	250	260
TOTAL	5,069	7,500
50 CHARGES AND OBLIGATIONS		
51 Rent	15,000	15,000
52 Insurance (Liability)	0	0
53 Dues, Memberships, & Subscriptions	150	390
54 Unclassified	0	0
TOTAL	15,150	15,390

PROFESSIONAL, PERSONNEL, AND OTHER EXPENDITURES		
10 Personnel Services (see attached)	$281,938	$369,495
20 Contractual Services	24,328	52,392
30 Supplies	4,195	3,200
40 Equipment	5,069	7,500
50 Charges and Obligations	15,150	15,390
TOTAL	$330,680	$447,977

*Inpatient program was 100% local funds, in addition to state-local shared funding of Comprehensive Mental Health Program.

Section A 10-Personnel Services (Administrative Services)	Current Program	Requested
Position No. from Table D — POSITION TITLE	(A) Year Ending June 30, 1978	(B) Year Ending June 30, 1979
1 — Executive Director	$23,580	$23,080
2 — Evaluation Coordinator	0	14,400
3 — Administrator Coordinator	13,450	15,420
4 — Account Clerk II	0	6,144
5 — Secretary III	6,978	7,992
6 — Clerk Typist II	4,464	5,748
CLIENT WAGES	0	0
Fringe Benefits	4,363	5,818
10-PERSONNEL SERVICES TOTAL	$52,835	$78,602

Section A 10-Personnel Services (Mental Health Services)	Current Program	Requested
Position No. from Table D — POSITION TITLE	(A) Year Ending June 30, 1978	(B) Year Ending June 30, 1979
1 — Program Director	$20,400	$20,000
2 — Medical Director	29,640	31,710
* 3 — M.H. Coordinator	0	6,600
4 — Supervisor II	15,120	16,680
5 — Psychiatrist	28,200	30,360
6 — Psychologist	16,435	13,500
7 — Social Worker I	5,328	10,452
8 — Social Worker I	8,880	10,416
9 — Social Worker I	4,440	5,064
10 — Crisis Intervention Counselor	0	12,000
11 — Crisis Intervention Counselor	0	12,000
12 — Supervisor I	11,920	13,700
13 — M.H. Teacher II	10,434	11,280
14 — Supervisor II	13,200	13,550
15 — M.H. Counselor I	8,088	9,628
16 — M.H. Teacher I	8,080	10,960
*17 — Vol. Services Liaison	7,654	9,288
18 — M.H. Nurse I	4,046	4,236
19 — Day Care Coordinator	11,760	13,350
20 — M.H. Assistant	2,943	5,526
21 — Community Liaison	11,440	12,500
22 — M.H. Nurse II	8,392	10,470
23 — M.H. Counselor I	0	8,880
24 — M.H. Counselor I	0	8,880
25 — Secretary IV	7,368	8,216
26 — Clerk Typist II	5,789	6,259
27 — Clerk Typist II	5,789	5,869
28 — Clerk Typist II	5,789	6,023
29 — Clerk Typist I	0	4,896
30 — Custodial Worker II	5,259	6,034
31 — Custodial Worker II	2,444	2,558
Program Summer Employment	0	600
Fringe Benefits	23,100	28,010
10-PERSONNEL SERVICES TOTAL	$281,938	$369,495

*Part-time jobs in 1978, combined into 1 job in 1979 budget.

Section A 10-Personnel Services (Aftercare Services)		Current Program	Requested
Position No. from Table D	POSITION TITLE	(A) Year Ending June 30, 1978	(B) Year Ending June 30, 1979
1	M.H. Supervisor II	$16,680	$16,680
2	Social Worker I	5,816	6,077
3	Social Worker I	3,877	4,051
	CLIENT WAGES	0	0
	Fringe Benefits	1,789	1,814
10-PERSONNEL SERVICES TOTAL		$28,162	$28,622

Section A 10-Personnel Services (Drug Program)		Current Program	Requested
Position No. from Table D	POSITION TITLE	(A) Year Ending June 30, 1978	(B) Year Ending June 30, 1979
1	Program Director	$21,000	$20,880
2	Treatment & Training Supvr. II	14,500	14,400
3	Counselor I	0	9,084
4	Clerk-Typist II	0	5,616
	CLIENT WAGES	0	
	Fringe Benefits	2,371	3,984
10-PERSONNEL SERVICES TOTAL		$37,871	53,964

DRUG PROGRAM - PERSONNEL AND OTHER EXPENSES

PROFESSIONAL, PERSONNEL, AND OTHER EXPENDITURES		
10 Personnel Services	$37,871	$53,964
20 Contractual Services	0	4,700
30 Supplies	0	900
40 Equipment	0	1,150
50 Charges and Obligations	5,000	3,125
TOTAL	$42,871	$63,839

EXHIBIT 2   NORTHERN DISTRICT STATE HOSPITAL

APPROPRIATION SUMMARY
(Requests vs Legislative Appropriations)

BIENNIUM COMPARISON	General Fund	Special Fund	Total Appropriations	
Operating Expenses:				
Requests 1976-78	$23,677,700	$7,727,800	$31,405,500	(75.4% G.F.)
Approp. 1974-76	$18,067,360	$6,241,050	$24,308,410	(74.3% G.F.)
Incr./(Decr.)	$ 5,610,340	$1,486,750	$ 7,097,090	
	% 31.1	% 23.8	% 29.2	
Capital Outlays:				
Approp. 1972-74	$ 1,862,970	$ 280,000	$ 2,142,970	
Approp. 1974-76	$ 208,300		$ 208,300	
Requests 1976-78	$ 3,750,780		$ 3,750,780	
Requests 1978-80	$ 1,485,000		$ 1,485,000	
Requests 1980-82	$ 1,045,000		$ 1,045,000	

ANNUAL APPROPRIATIONS FOR OPERATING EXPENSES

	General Fund	Special Fund	Total Appropriations
Approp. 1974-75	$ 9,118,795	$3,029,075	$12,147,870
Incr./(Decr.)	$ 1,549,935	$ (50,370)	$ 1,499,565
vs. 1973-74	% 20.5	% (1.6)	% 14.1
Approp. 1975-76	$ 8,948,565	$3,211,975	$12,160,540
Incr./(Decr.)	$ (170,230)	$ 182,900	12,670
vs. 1974-75	% (1.9)	% 6.0	0.1
Requests 1976-77	$11,793,340	$3,738,700	$15,532,040
Incr./(Decr.)	$ 2,844,775	$ 526,725	$ 3,371,500
vs. 1975-76	% 31.8	% 16.4	% 27.7
Requests 1977-78	$11,884,360	$3,989,100	$15,873,460
Incr./(Decr.)	$ 91,020	$ 250,400	$ 341,420
vs. 1976-77	% 0.8	% 6.7	% 2.2

BUDGET COMPONENTS--ADMINISTRATION

	Appropriations 1975-1976	Requested 1976-1977	1977-1978
1100 Personnel Services	$437,940	$539,435	$565,335
1110 Salaries, classified positions	441,230	538,655	564,975
1111 Salaries, overtime	0	2,500	2,500
1120 Wages (temporary personnel)	6,900	6,900	6,900
1150 Patient labor	840	0	0
Less: For turnover and vacancies (1.6%)	-11,030	-8,620	-9,040
1200 Contractual Services	$ 72,305	$121,475	$123,085
1210 General repairs (100 service calls @ $20)		2,400	2,600
1211 Maintenance service contracts (2 scales @ $6)	12	15	15
1213 Professional services		3,860	4,430
1214 Travel - convention and education		545	545
1243 Travel - mileage		4,950	4,950
1246 Travel - subsistence and lodging		1,505	1,505
1261 Postal service		11,465	11,635
1262 Messenger service		240	240
1265 Telecommunications		93,095	93,095
1270 Printing and other office services		360	390
1300 Supplies and Materials	$ 8,250	$ 16,305	$ 17,660
1340 Office supplies		15,200	16,465
1380 Educational and recreational supplies		100	105
1391 Motor vehilce supplies		950	1,030
1500 Equipment - Replacement	$ 1,700	$ 9,755	0
1510 Office equipment		8,905	0
1599 Other equipment (warehouse)		850	0
1600 Equipment - Additional		$ 1,045	0
1610 Office equipment		1,045	0
1700 Current Charges and Obligations	$ 6,290	$ 15,510	$ 16,595
1731 Rent (business equipment)		7,150	7,750
1742 Insurance (workmen's compensation)		40	45
1743 Insurance (surety)		35	40
1749 Insurance (liability)		880	915
1789 Dues and subscriptions		1,690	1,830
1791 Unemployment compensation		2,130	2,130
1794 Workmen's compensation awards		3,585	3,885
1900 Recoveries	-$ 8,000	-$ 6,480	-$ 7,020
TOTAL OPERATING EXPENSES	$518,485	$697,045	$715,655

BUDGET COMPONENTS--CARE AND TREATMENT OF PATIENTS

	Appropriations 1975-1976	Requested 1976-1977	1977-1978
1100 Personnel Services	$7,813,760	$ 9,358,500	$ 9,808,310
1100 Salaries, classified positions	$8,161,725	$ 9,335,955	$ 9,792,160
(new positions requested)			
3 psychiatrists			
1 physician			
20 mental health technicians			
1 occupational therapy director			
1 pharmacist			
3 psychiatric social workers			
1 psychologist			
6 special activities assistants			
1111 Salaries, overtime	0	3,260	3,260
1120 Wages (temporary)	29,795	41,600	41,600
1150 Patient labor	19,000	0	0
Less: Turnover and vacancies	$ 391,760	$ 288,050	$ 301,960
(3% of classified positions)			
1200 Contractual Services	$ 75,360	$ 173,675	$ 180,180
1210 General repairs		10,200	11,050
1211 Maintenance services contracts		770	830
1213 Professional services (x-ray)		360	390
1214 Health professional services		36,395	39,305
1215 Hospital services		60,565	61,560
1217 Clinic services		940	1,015
1218 Laboratory and x-ray		43,950	45,990
1241 Travel - convention		3,885	3,380
1243 Travel - mileage		11,275	11,195
1246 Travel - subsistence and lodging		700	700
1251 Freight services		385	415
1270 Printing and other office supplies			
1290 Agency service contracts		770	770
1299 Other contractual services		2,010	2,180
1300 Supplies and Materials	$ 422,650	$ 527,945	$ 554,845
1340 Office supplies		31,030	33,620
1350 Drugs		210,330	218,560
1351 Medical appliances		215	235
1352 Dental supplies		1,370	1,315
1355 Medical and laboratory supplies		91,250	94,610
1370 Housekeeping supplies		95,020	102,940
1380 Educational supplies		9,160	9,770
1393 Patient's wearing apparel		62,245	67,430
1394 Employees' wearing apparel		17,025	15,205
1399 Other supplies		10,300	11,160

	Appropriations 1975-1976	Requested 1976-1977	1977-1978
1500 Equipment - Replacement	$ 14,205	$ 133,860	$ 0
1510 Office equipment		30,140	0
1520 Household equipment		94,595	0
1530 Medical and laboratory equipment		7,485	0
1571 Recreational equipment		1,045	0
1596 Photographic equipment		595	0
1600 Equipment - Additional	0	75,340	8,035
1610 Office equipment		11,995	1,920
1620 Household equipment		10,585	6,115
1630 Medical and laboratory equipment		49,745	0
1670 Educational equipment		300	0
1671 Recreational equipment		490	0
1696 Photographic equipment		1,375	0
1697 Electronic equipment		350	0
1699 Other equipment		500	0
1700 Current Charges and Obligations	$ 26,425	$ 87,790	$ 94,540
1731 Rent (business equipment)		6,990	7,575
1742 Insurance (workmen's compensation)		690	720
1743 Insurance (surety)		155	170
1749 Insurance (liability)		17,910	18,855
1789 Dues and subscriptions		3,585	3,885
1791 Unemployment compensation		10,800	11,700
1794 Workmen's compensation awards		44,280	47,970
1799 Other current charges		3,380	3,665
TOTAL OPERATING EXPENSES	$8,352,400	$10,357,110	$10,645,910

NORTHERN DISTRICT STATE HOSPITAL

BUDGET COMPONENTS--SUPPORT SERVICES

		Appropriations 1975-1976	Requested	
			1976-1977	1977-1978
1.	Operation of laundry (49 employees)	$ 251,805	$ 323,355	$ 336,350
2.	Operation of power plant	$ 338,085	$ 593,005	$ 596,685
3.	Maintenance of building and grounds	$ 869,460	$1,456,290	$1,394,705
4.	Contractual services (consultation and education)	$ 148,065	$ 167,945	$ 174,845
5.	Food service	$1,589,120	$1,816,490	$1,879,040
6.	Employees' cafeteria	$ 93,120	$ 97,890	$ 105,425
7.	Electronic data processing	0	$ 22,920	$ 24,845
		$3,289,655	$4,477,895	$4,511,895

FRAME III

CONTINGENCY PLANNING

You are the director of the Tri-County Mental Health Center.
In attempting to develop next year's budget, you know that you must do
contingency planning. Since the budget itself is already written, you
now need to plan for the things that might go wrong. You are looking
for all possible changes and anticipating how you would deal with those
budgetary changes. Anticipatory planning is a crucial aspect of good
budget management.

Step 1. Individual Planning (5 minutes)

On the following pages are each of the things that you think might
go wrong. Within your group, have each member choose a number from 1
to 6. Be sure that all numbers from 1 to 6 are taken. Work on the
contingency item that corresponds to the number you have chosen. Read
it to yourself and then decide what you would do, based on your
understanding of the mental health center budget.

Take no more than 5 minutes to complete this step. When each of
you has finished working on his/her contingency item, move to the next
step.

Step 2. Group Sharing (25 minutes)

Start with Contingency Item #1. Have the person who worked on
that item read to the group and give the response that he/she
formulated in Step 1. Each of you has approximately 4 minutes to read
and give your response to the contingency item.

Contingency Item #1

The latest rumor from the state capital is that an 8% reduction in current operating budgets could be required of all agencies receiving state funds within the next budget year, due to anticipated reduced state revenues. Your mental health center receives 60% of its funding from the state.

Assuming the worst eventuality (that you must cut your state share by 8%) which program area(s) could contribute to the 8% reduction?

Contingency Item #2

The County Commission provides approximately 3% of your funding. Next year is an election year. You are aware that there has been pressure from the community for services to meet the geriatric mental health needs of nursing home and boarding home residents. One of your sources in the County Commission staff has told you that you might have some capital expenditure funds diverted to your Center, so that you would end up with 5% more money than you had last year. You also are well aware that the staff of your center has not received a pay raise in two years, and morale is slipping.

How would you spend the extra 5%?

Contingency Item #3

At a recent staff meeting, your staff indicated a need for more in-service training since many new problem cases were being referred to the Center (alcoholics, suicide attempts, and drug dependent elementary school children) for which very few staff had any expertise. If this increase in new problem cases continues, would you reallocate funds for special training? If so, which funds?

Contingency Item #4

Efforts have been made to unionize the clerical and custodial staff at the Center. The unionization may become a reality next year. If that happens, you know that one of their very first demands will be an immediate pay raise of at least 10%. Where in the budget could you find the money?

Contingency Item #5

You have received a call from the regional office of the National Institute of Mental Health indicating that 8% of your budget is not in compliance with the federal staffing grant. Staffing funds were inappropriately used to buy typewriters and desks, which is an error that you did not know your fiscal officer had made. Since you must make up this 8% error somewhere, where will you locate the funds?

Contingency Item #6

The legislature may pass an alcoholism rehabilitation act during their next session. This act would require that all intoxicated persons who are picked up by the police be taken to the local mental health center rather than be incarcerated. You estimate that this act would cost your Center $15,000. In the past, the legislature has provided you with only about 75% of what you have requested. The County Commission has provided you with about 90% of what you have requested. For example, if you request $10,000 from the state, you are likely to receive $7,500. Similarly, if you ask for $5,000 from the county, you are likely to receive $4,500, and as a result, you are $3,000 short ($2,500 + $500). Given the $15,000 you must get from some source, and given your past record with both the legislature and the County Commission, how will you make up the shortage if this act passes?

FRAME IV

COSTING OUT SERVICES

You decide as superintendent of Northern District State Hospital that more attention is needed in the area of costing out hospital treatment services in order to prepare for program budgeting. You will start with the program that deals with geriatric patients. In reviewing the budget, you will note that patient per-diem costs as well as other unit costs are already computed ($23.65 per patient per day).

Since 40% of your residents are geriatric patients, you have decided to call a staff meeting with representatives of the geriatric nursing service, social service, medical service, recreational service, and financial management office.

Patient Care Information

Psychiatric Patients under 65 comprise 55% of the average population, but represent about 85% of admissions. Of these, approximately 410 suffer from active forms of mental disorder and substance abuse, 145 are in advanced stages of chronic mental illness, and 239 are able to participate in social and community activities on a controlled basis.

Geriatric Patients (65 and over) comprise 40% of the average population, but only about 15% of admissions. Of these, approximately 90 receive intensive care in a certified unit, 240 require continued treatment because of their severely chronic condition, and 270 are in intermediate care in a certified unit.

Medical-Surgical Patients comprise 5% of the population and are admitted from the above groups for general hospital care, whether related or not to their mental illness.

1. Average Population by Program

Program	1974-75	1975-76	1976-77	1977-78
Geriatric (65 and over)				
Intensive Treatment (Medicaid Certified)	90	85	80	80
Continued Treatment	240	245	175	165
Intermediate Care (Medicaid Certified)	270	270	230	220
Total	600	600	485	465

2. Patient Day Cost Factor

	Total expense	Patient days	Cost per patient day
1972-73	$10,258,489	790,955	12.97
1973-74	11,740,227	617,945	19.00
1974-75	12,552,868	530,710	23.65
1975-76 (Appropriated)	12,160,540	530,700	22.74
1976-77 (Requested)	15,434,150	456,250	33.83
1977-78 (Requested)	15,768,035	438,000	36.00

Step 1. Budget Calculations (10 minutes)

Working in groups of two, review the budget in order to calculate all the costs for administration and supportive services that affect 40% of the patients for 1975-76. Then calculate all personnel costs for this patient population and divide by the number of patients in order to arrive at your per-diem patient care and treatment costs.

_____

_____

_____

_____

_____

_____

_____

_____

Step 2. Program Budget Preparation (20 minutes)

The superintendent reconvenes all service representatives to share their calculations on patient treatment costs. Once consensus is reached on the unit cost, the staff meeting discussion shifts to the specification of program objectives and output in which annual patient treatment costs are divided up among program objectives.

The instructor should assign the following general roles which will not be defined: superintendent, nursing representatives, social service representatives, medical service representatives, recreation program representatives, and financial management office representatives. The staff as a whole should jointly contribute to the development of the following budget profile:

PROGRAM OBJECTIVES FOR GERIATRIC PATIENTS	PORTION OF ANNUAL PATIENT TREATMENT COSTS	OUTPUTS/BENEFITS PER PROGRAM OBJECTIVE
1.		
2.		
3.		
4.		
5.		

Step 3. Budget Alternatives (20 minutes)

The superintendent has just learned that in the next legislative session all budget presentations must show alternative costs for providing the same level of care in the community. While patient treatment costs were calculated and programmatically defined in the previous frame, all supportive services should now be calculated per patient annually. To simplify the process, each simulation participant should total the entire budget for 1975-76 (administration, care and treatment, and support), multiply it by .4 for the 40% geriatric population, subtract the total patient treatment costs for all geriatric patients annually (calculated in prior frame) and this will yield the total supportive service costs.

The superintendent has called another staff meeting with the same service representatives. The first item on the agenda is to reach consensus on the annual supportive service costs for the geriatric patients at Northern District State Hospital.

With the patient treatment costs and the supportive service costs, all the service representatives should complete the following cost comparison activity based on the recent information that geriatric patients could be placed in nursing homes ($550 per month per patient) with special treatment services provided by the local community mental health center ($200 per month per patient).

(More of this step appears on the following two pages.)

STATE HOSPITAL (ANNUAL)

Patient Treatment Services	Cost Per Patient	Total Cost For All Geriatric Patients
1.		
2.		
3.		
4.		

Supportive Services

    Food, shelter, clothing, etc.

Total Cost $_____

NURSING HOME (ANNUAL)

Patient Treatment Services	Cost Per Patient	Total Cost For All Geriatric Patients
	$200/month X 12	
Supportive Services	$500/month X 12	

Total Cost $_____

Once these comparative costs have been developed, consensus should be reached on the calculations and on the relative cost benefit for services provided in the state hospital in contrast to the community. For the purpose of this simulation, the issue of relocating the geriatric patient in the community in terms of social costs (confusion and disorientation) and physical costs (potential deterioration and death) should not be considered in the decision making. What recommendations should the superintendent take with him/her when he/she is called to testify before the legislature on the next year's budget? What is your rationale for that decision?

_____

_____

_____

_____

_____

_____

_____

_____

_____

_____

_____

_____

FRAME V

DEBRIEFING

(20 minutes)

While this simulation has included a number of calculations, the primary objective was to refine budget analysis skills.

1. What are some of the significant differences between a state hospital and community mental health center budget?

2. Does the size of the agency have any relationship to budgetary considerations?

3. What are some of the problems in doing contingency planning?

4. What are some of the assumptions which are made in costing out services which are part of a larger agency like a state hospital?

5. Which do you think provides more accountability, program or line-item budgeting? Why?

REFERENCES

Howard, S. K. Changing state budgeting. Lexington, Ky.: Council of State Governments, 1973.

RELATED READINGS

Cooper, E. M. Guidelines for a minimum statistical and accounting system for community mental health centers. Rockville, Md.: National Institute of Mental Health, 1977.

Hatry, H. P., Winnie, R. E., & Fisk, D. M. Practical program evaluation for state and local government officials. Washington, D. C.: The Urban Institute, 1973.

Perloff, H. S., & Nathan, R. P. Revenue sharing and the city. Baltimore: The Johns Hopkins Press, 1968.

Rivlin, A. M. Systematic thinking for social action. Washington, D. C.: The Brookings Institute, 1971.

Schultz, C. L. The politics and economics of public spending. Washington, D. C.: The Brookings Institute, 1968.

Sorensen, J. E., & Phipps, D. W. Cost-finding and rate-setting for community mental health centers. Rockville, Md.: National Institute of Mental Health, 1975.

Sze, W. C., & Hopps, J. C. (Eds.). Evaluation and accountability in human service programs. Cambridge, Mass.: Schenkman Publishing Co., Inc., 1974.

Turnbull, A. B., III. Governmental budgeting and PPBS: A programmed introduction. Reading, Mass.: Addison-Wesley Publishing Co., 1970.

5

GRIEVANCE

I. <u>INTRODUCTION</u>

The purpose of this simulation is to acquaint participants with
the skills and procedures necessary to handle effectively employees'
complaints about their jobs (relationships with peers, nature and
amount of work, relationship with supervisor, etc.). It is only
natural that someone, at some time, will be dissatisfied with some
aspect of his/her work. This dissatisfaction or complaint is not
necessarily a grievance. The term "grievance" has a rather specific
connotation in labor relations. It refers to a document completed by
an employee which indicates the employee's discontent with some aspect
of his/her job. The effective manager obviously seeks to avoid or
prevent situations which could lead to grievances. However, if
grievances are filed, a supervisor or administrator must know how to
attain or retain good employee-supervisor relationships while
protecting management's (or the agency's) interests.

The key to handling complaints and/or grievances satisfactorily
lies initially, and most importantly, with the employee's immediate
supervisor. That supervisor must listen carefully to what the
employee is saying, make certain he/she has the facts straight, deal
with the complaint in a manner which is consistent with the
organization's policies and practices, and explain all actions taken
or not taken to the employee. A model for this most crucial aspect of
handling grievances is provided in Frame I of this simulation.

Grievances may be filed in both union and non-union organizations.
Generally speaking, a unionized organization has precise regulations

which state who must do what, and by when. Non-unionized organizations, and particularly smaller organizations, may have a grievance process set up in a more informal manner. Yet for union or non-union organizations the general procedure for handling grievances remains the same. The organization must clearly define "grievance" in terms of the legitimate grounds for filing a grievance. The employee must do certain things in order to file a grievance. In most organizations, this means filling out a form which includes at least the date, the employee's name, and a statement of the grievance. The employee and the immediate supervisor then confer. The immediate supervisor decides either to grant or to deny the grievance. The employee may file an appeal if the immediate supervisor's decision did not remedy the situation to the employee's satisfaction. A higher level supervisor (division head, department head, agency head, etc.) reviews the grievance and renders a decision. If still dissatisfied with the decision, the employee can usually file an appeal with an outside source of authority (the state personnel agency, the court, a federal agency such as the Equal Employment Opportunity Commission). Definite time limits are generally established for hearings, filing of appeals, and rendering decisions.

In every agency, regardless of its size, all employees must be familiar with the grievance procedure and their rights under this procedure. They should have copies of the written policies concerning grievances and the necessary forms readily available to them (i.e., securing forms without going through a supervisor or management person). Management at all levels must be equally acquainted with the policies and forms and, in addition, must be well versed in how to handle grievances.

If you are a manager, having a grievance filed against you does not mean that you are the worst supervisor in the agency. On the contrary! A good manager should expect grievances. If you have too many filed against you, then the employees and you are not communicating as well as you should. From an employee's point of view, filing a grievance is generally a big step. Many times, the complaint or dissatisfaction can be worked out to please both of you before the grievance stage is reached.

A few general principles and reminders about managers and grievances are good to remember. Don't take a grievance filed by one of your employees as a personal insult to you. Sometimes the grievance concerns a policy or practice over which you have no control (such as an agency's policy on granting personal leave). In settling dissatisfactions or grievances, be consistent with both your own style of management and the organization's policies and procedures. Check with other managers in your organization to see what they've done and with the current revisions to official policy before making your own decision. Make certain you understand exactly the nature of the employee's problem. And make certain that you explain the reasoning behind your decision. Set a timetable for alleviation of the problem, and stick to it. Check up on how the solution is working for both you and the employee periodically. And, above all, remember that you are the person in the middle: you must represent your organization's interest and, at the same time, work on a day-to-day, face-to-face basis with employees who may or may not share your commitment to the organization.

II. GOAL AND ENABLING OBJECTIVES

Goal:

> To provide participants with the skills and knowledge needed to handle grievances as administrators or supervisors.

Enabling Objectives:

Upon completing this simulation, participants should:

1. Perform effectively in a supervisor-employee confrontation.

2. Know the critical components of a grievance procedure.

3. Know the general procedures followed in settling a grievance in a unionized setting.

4. Be able to serve as an effective witness for management in an arbitration hearing.

III. PROCEDURES

FRAME I - Employee-Supervisor Confrontation

      Step 1. Evaluating an Employee (10 minutes)
      Step 2. Sharing Evaluations (5 minutes)
      Step 3. Dealing Directly with an Employee's Dissatisfaction
              (20 minutes)
      Step 4. Debriefing (15 minutes)

FRAME II - Grievance Handling

      Step 1. Analyzing Grievances (10 minutes)
      Step 2. Defining Problems (10 minutes)
      Step 3. Sharing Problems and Formulating Solutions (20 minutes)
      Step 4. Evaluating Solutions (15 minutes)
      Step 5. Debriefing (10 minutes)

FRAME III - Handling Grievances in a Unionized Setting

      Step 1. Setting the Scene (5 minutes)
      Step 2. Sorting Out the Evidence (20 minutes)
      Step 3. Sharing Responses (10 minutes)
      Step 4. The Hearing (15 minutes)
      Step 5. Debriefing (10 minutes)

FRAME I

EMPLOYEE-SUPERVISOR CONFRONTATION

In this frame, participants will assume the role of a supervisor who must evaluate the performance of an employee. The participants will evaluate an employee's performance and then meet with that employee when the employee protests the evaluation. This protest is not yet a grievance, but it could become one. The effective supervisor resolves 70 to 80% of employees' dissatisfactions before they become formal, filed grievances.

Step 1. Evaluating an Employee (10 minutes)

You are Cynthia Fubar, the Assistant Director of the Rotterdam Community Mental Health Center. One of your responsibilities includes the records system and seeing that records are transferred to the appropriate offices and agencies as clients are moved through the mental health care system, from intake to treatment to follow-up to community readjustment. Thus, part of your job is essentially one of supervising paperwork--making certain that the file clerks under your supervision keep each client's file intact, deliver it to the appropriate persons at the appropriate times, retrieve the file, and refile it once it is returned to your office.

One of your file clerks is Wayne Floyd. He works full time for you and is also trying to go to college full time. Although you don't know him well, you do know that he often does not adequately attend to his work. It is time for his six months' evaluation. This evaluation will determine whether he will be kept on as an employee and whether he will receive a raise. You know you are the "person in the middle"--you must deal with Wayne on a day-to-day basis and you must remain loyal to management's responsibility of retaining competent and effective staff. On the following pages are: (1) your personal notes on his performance which reflect actual events and circumstances; (2) the mental health center's regulations concerning employee performance; and (3) his evaluation form.

Review the notes, read the regulations, and complete the evaluation form. Work individually. When all participants have finished their evaluations of Wayne Floyd, move on to the next step in this exercise.

1. PERSONAL NOTES ON WAYNE FLOYD - FILE CLERK I

January - Completed training. Has worked under Ruth Bennett, the woman with the most experience. She says that he does well when he pays attention, but his mind wanders quite a bit and then he "messes up."

February - Misplaced eight files, 2/9. Ruth and I found them in his desk after he left work on 2/10. Late 2/19, 2/23.

March - Day of personal leave granted, 3/15. Absent on 3/16, 3/17; did not phone in any of those days. Unable to reach him at home. Said he was sick when he returned. One day of sick leave and one day of annual leave granted, and reprimanded orally, upon his return. Late 3/18 and 3/19.

April - Sent to hospital to pick up records of clients being released to Rotterdam CMHC's Aftercare Program, 4/2. Returned two hours later, with county car's gas gauge on "empty." Said he got lost; next person using the car found library books checked out to him in the back seat. Late on 4/12, 4/19, and 4/25. Returned from lunch on 4/28 in what appeared to be intoxicated state; reprimanded orally.

May - Late 5/10, 5/20, and 5/24. Office unable to find 25 clients' records, 5/4. Ruth Bennett says they were assigned to him to file, but no sure way to substantiate this. Search of entire filing system requires 3 days; missing records located, 5/10. He grumbles about the monotony of hunting for them! Asks for annual leave on 5/26, 5/27, and 5/28, and was granted.

June - Absent from office on 6/15. After two hours, was found sleeping in men's rest room; reprimanded orally. Behind in his work week of 6/14-6/18; found reading textbooks in the file area three times. Late 6/8, 6/17, 6/21, and 6/25. Asks for promotion to File Clerk II and pay raise on 6/23.

ROTTERDAM COMMUNITY MENTAL HEALTH CENTER
EMPLOYEE REGULATIONS
DISCIPLINE SCHEDULE

Event	First Offense	Second Offense	Third Offense
Absenteeism	Oral or Written Reprimand	Written Reprimand or 3 days' suspension	3 days' suspension or dismissal
Insubordination	Oral Reprimand	Written Reprimand	3 days' suspension
Dress and Grooming	Oral Reprimand	Oral or Written Reprimand	Written Reprimand or 3 days' suspension
Fights & Altercations	Written Reprimand	5 days' suspension	Dismissal
Abusing Clients	Written Reprimand	Written Reprimand or 5 days' suspension	5 days' suspension or dismissal
Intoxication & Alcoholism	Oral or Written Reprimand	Written Reprimand or 1 day's suspension	3 days' suspension or dismissal
Off-Duty Misconduct	Written Reprimand	Written Reprimand or 3 days' suspension	3 days suspension or dismissal
Sleeping & Loafing	Oral Reprimand	Written Reprimand	1 day's suspension
Dishonesty	Oral Reprimand	Written Reprimand	1 day's suspension
Abuse or Mis-Use of Agency Property	Oral or Written Reprimand	Written Reprimand or 3 days' suspension	3 days' suspension or dismissal
Tardiness	Oral Reprimand	Written Reprimand	1 day's suspension
Incompetence	Oral or Written Reprimand	Written Reprimand or 3 days' suspension	3 days' suspension or dismissal
Carelessness	Oral Reprimand	Written Reprimand	1 day's suspension

ROTTERDAM COMMUNITY MENTAL HEALTH CENTER

PERSONNEL EVALUATION FORM

Date _July 1_

Type of Evaluation

_✓_ Six months

_____ Yearly

Employee's Name _Wayne Floyd_ Position _File Clerk I_

Length of time employed by RCMHC _6 mo._; in your section _6 mo._

EVALUATION (CHECK ONE BOX PER ITEM)

	POOR	FAIR	GOOD	EXCELLENT
Personal Appearance				
Initiative				
Attitude				
Quality of Work Completed				
Quantity of Work Completed				
Potential				
Relations with Other Employees				

Recommended Disposition of this Employee:

_____ Dismissed

_____ Kept on probation for another _____ months

_____ Granted permanent civil service status

_____ Granted permanent civil service status and given raise of ____ %

_____ Granted permanent civil service status and promoted to _____

Cynthia Julay
Signature

asst Dir., RCMHC.
Position

Step 2. Sharing Evaluations (5 minutes)

Divide into subgroups of three, four, or five persons each. Compare your evaluations of Wayne Floyd. In particular, what was your recommended disposition of him?

Now decide among yourselves what your group's evaluation of him would be. That is, come to consensus on your rating of his personal appearance, initiative, etc., and agree upon a recommended disposition for him. Record your group's consensus on the evaluation form below so that you can use it for the next step.

When your small group has completed this task, proceed to the next step.

EVALUATION (CHECK ONE BOX PER ITEM)

	POOR	FAIR	GOOD	EXCELLENT
Personal Appearance				
Initiative				
Attitude				
Quality of Work Completed				
Quantity of Work Completed				
Potential				
Relations with Other Employees				

Disposition _____

Step 3. Dealing Directly with an Employee's Dissatisfaction
(20 minutes)

Cynthia Fubar knows Wayne Floyd is going to be upset when he sees his personnel evaluation. She goes to the Director of the Center and receives the following "pointers" for dealing with Wayne (Patterson & Snyder, 1975):

- let the employee tell his/her story;

- adopt a problem-solving attitude;

- don't take the complaint or grievance personally;

- ask only objective questions;

- give full attention to the employee (i.e., accept no phone calls during the time you are meeting);

- after employee has finished speaking, go over his/her story again and write down specific parts and the specific remedy that he/she is seeking;

- restate employee's own story in your own words and check with employee to see if it is correct;

- set an appointment (date and time) for the next meeting, in which you will tell him/her your decision.

Within your group, choose one person to play the role of Wayne Floyd. Choose another person to be Cynthia Fubar. The remaining persons will be observers, who will report on the interaction that will take place.

Assume that Wayne Floyd has received his evaluation and notice of his disposition (that is, dismissed, kept on probation, retained, given a raise, or promoted). He is upset by the evaluation and has come to Ms. Fubar to discuss the matter.

The person assuming the role of Wayne Floyd should turn to the page entitled "Role Play Instructions for Wayne Floyd" and read only that page. The person assuming the role of Cynthia Fubar should turn to the page entitled "Role Play Instructions for Cynthia Fubar" and read only that page. Observers should turn to the page entitled "Instructions for Observers" and read only that page.

When all participants have read their appropriate pages, begin the role play in which Wayne Floyd confronts his supervisor about his evaluation. Complete the role play in 15 minutes and then proceed to the next step.

Role Play Instructions for <u>Wayne Floyd</u>

You had thought you were doing a pretty good job as a file clerk, considering how dull the job is and how the pressures of school have been getting to you. You are angry about the evaluation, but you also want to keep your job. Without your job, you cannot get through school.

You had told Ms. Fubar when you applied for the job that you were going to be in school, and you had gotten the distinct impression that you would be supported in your schooling efforts. You assumed that work time could be made up around examination time (March and June) and that some tardiness was O.K.

You have just found out that the Rotterdam Community Mental Health Center has a "Discipline Schedule," which you saw only yesterday. It was not given to you when you were first employed. You see clearly that you could have received one day's suspension for the third time you were late. Had you known the RCHMC was so strict about tardiness, you certainly would have been on time every day. You think that, since you were not informed about this discipline schedule, you should not be held responsible for your lateness.

What you want to get out of this meeting with your supervisor is a revised evaluation, one which will grant you at least permanent civil service status. You desperately need a raise, and you truly feel that you deserve it.

Role Play Instructions for <u>Cynthia Fubar</u>

Like most people, you really hate face-to-face confrontations with people, especially when you must work with them every day.

In relation to Wayne Floyd, you feel that you have been more than patient and tolerant with him. Despite the "Discipline Schedule," you have not suspended him for being tardy. It is difficult to believe the number of times that he has been tardy. He knew the penalty for lateness. And you were even more shocked when he had the nerve to ask for a raise! You know he needs the job to stay in school--and you also know that you need a much more dependable stream of work from him if you are to do your job properly.

In sum, you like Wayne as a person, but he has not been a particularly good employee. You will stand by your evaluation and try to help him understand the problem.

Instructions for <u>Observers</u>

Watch the interaction between the two players carefully. At the completion of the role play, you should have written down the answers to the following questions:

1. Did Ms. Fubar really listen to Wayne? _____

   Did she repeat in her own words what he had said? _____

2. Did the two people come to an agreement on exactly what the

   problem is? _____

   Was the problem adequately defined to the satisfaction of both

   persons? _____

3. Did Ms. Fubar ask Wayne what he felt would be an appropriate

   solution to his grievance? _____

4. Did Ms. Fubar try to get all the facts? _____

5. Did Ms. Fubar present her side of the story? _____

6. Did anyone make reference to official policies of the RCMHC?

   _____

   If so, who did? _____

   To what did they refer? _____

7. Did Ms. Fubar:

   _____ give her decision immediately at the end of the meeting, or

   _____ promise to tell him of her decision at some unspecified time,

   or

   _____ promise to tell him of her decision at a definite future time

   and place?

Step 4. Debriefing (15 minutes)

Staying in your small groups, answer the following questions:

1. Let the observers give their reactions to the role play between Wayne Floyd and Cynthia Fubar. How well did the supervisor-employee interaction concerning a dissatisfaction or grievance follow the principles noted in the beginning of Step 3? What did Ms. Fubar do well? What did she do poorly?

2. Do you think Wayne Floyd will file a grievance?

3. How much does a supervisor's liking or disliking of an employee play a part in his/her evaluation of that employee?

4. Do you think that the RCMHC's "Discipline Schedule" is realistic? Do you think that such detailed description of offenses and punishments is necessary?

5. How does size of an organization effect the formality or informality of its personnel procedures?

FRAME II

GRIEVANCE HANDLING

In this frame, participants will serve as consultants who define problems and formulate solutions for certain situations which relate to handling grievances.

Step 1. Analyzing Grievances (10 minutes)

You work for the State Division of Personnel. Within the last two months, all state employees have been granted the right to bargain collectively. Since the passage of collective bargaining legislation, you have been very busy, visiting different state institutions to explain the new rules and regulations to management and employees. You have also been serving as a consultant to the management of these institutions, helping them with the various procedures that can be covered under collective bargaining (such as the handling of grievances).

This week you are at Brooksville State Hospital, which is the state's largest institution. It does not have a union. Today, at the request of the Superintendent, you are working with Barbara Jackson, who is the 52-year-old white director of Social Services at the hospital. She reports to the assistant superintendent for Clinical Services. On the staff of Social Services and under her direct supervision are 13 social workers who are assigned to various units throughout the hospital. Two of her social workers are assigned to each of the following units: Adult Male, Adult Female, Geriatric, Alcoholic, Forensic, and Adolescent. One social worker is assigned to the Intake Unit.

Until a month ago, Ms. Jackson felt that her department was running quite smoothly. Recently two grievances have been filed and she is uncertain about the best method to handle them.

The first grievance was filed by Chuck Wheeler, a 24-year-old black social worker who has been employed at Brooksville State Hospital for two months. Chuck's specialty in his M.S.W. program was gerontology. His assignment at the hospital has been to the

Adolescent Unit, however. Chuck filed a grievance against Ms. Jackson over his work assignment, claiming that he was promised the Geriatric Unit during his job interview with Ms. Jackson but was arbitrarily and capriciously given the Adolescent Unit on his first day of work. He further claims that the assignment was a racist act. To document this last contention, Chuck notes in his grievance that the patient population on the Geriatric Unit is only 46% black, while the Adolescent Unit is 52% black. He is now threatening to file a complaint against Ms. Jackson and the hospital with the Equal Employment Opportunity Commission. Since filing the grievance, Chuck has, in Ms. Jackson's opinion, not been performing well at all. He has been late to Social Services staff meetings several times without offering any kind of reason, has neglected to fill out reports properly, and has not assumed a caseload that is in any way commensurate with that of the other social worker assigned to the unit.

You ask Ms. Jackson if she did in fact promise him the Geriatric Unit. She replies emphatically that she did not; what she did promise him was to try to move him to the Geriatric Unit when and if one of the other social workers, all of whom have seniority over Chuck, resigned and shuffling of assignments then became necessary. She told you that because Chuck has not yet worked for the state for six months, he is still on probation. All the other social workers under her direction are permanent members of the State Civil Service system, having completed their six months' probationary period satisfactorily. Therefore, she feels it would not be proper to move another social worker to another unit against that person's will, just to satisfy Chuck. Two other social workers are black in addition to Chuck, and they have made no complaint that she knows of either about their assignment or about racism on her part.

You then ask Ms. Jackson what she is doing now with Chuck, in view of her opinion of his performance on the job. She tells you she has been working with Chuck, talking to him in an effort to understand why he feels that racism is the cause of his work assignment. She thinks he might still harbor some hostility from his university days, when he attended a predominantly white institution of higher education. She thinks that if she can reduce his hostility, he will be more willing to become a "member of the team." She is thinking of asking the other two black social workers to talk to Chuck about this, and she wants to know what you think of that idea.

The second grievance was filed by the two social workers on her staff who are assigned to the Forensic Unit. Their grievance centers on their salaries. Although they receive salaries commensurate with the other social workers of Social Services, they claim that they should be entitled to hazardous duty pay due to their assignment to the Forensic Unit. Other employees who spend the majority of their day working on the Forensic Unit (psychiatric aides, nurses, etc.) receive this hazardous duty pay, but they do not. State regulations specifically exclude social workers, psychiatrists, psychologists, and medical doctors from those eligible for hazardous duty pay. Their grievance was filed against the unit head of the Forensic Unit, not against Ms. Jackson. Since filing their grievance, they have taken up much of the Social Services' staff meeting time talking about their grievance, according to Ms. Jackson. In contrast to Chuck Wheeler, however, Ms. Jackson feels that they have continued to perform their duties as well as they did prior to the filing of the grievance.

You ask Ms. Jackson exactly what the problem is. Although she finds it hard to put into words, she feels that somehow the "feeling" or the "quality" of her relations with her staff has gone down. When the two social workers from the Forensic Unit begin to talk about how unjust the salary differential is, their colleagues agree with them. The result is that staff meetings often become prolonged sessions of "Ain't it awful!" rather than productive sessions in which other problems are resolved.

Step 2. Defining Problems (10 minutes)

Divide into groups of two and work with your partner to evaluate the grievances in the prior step in order to identify clearly the problems which exist in Social Services at Brooksville State Hospital. On the lines below, write out what each problem is and cite the evidence to support your definition of that problem. There can be from one to three problems per grievance. The problems can reside in the procedures used for handling grievances, in the structure of the hospital, or in Ms. Jackson's involvement with the persons making the grievances. Define the problems which you see in each grievance.

CHUCK WHEELER'S GRIEVANCE   FORENSIC UNIT'S GRIEVANCE

Problem _____   Problem _____

_____   _____

Evidence _____   Evidence _____

_____   _____

Problem _____   Problem _____

_____   _____

Evidence _____   Evidence _____

_____   _____

Problem _____   Problem _____

_____   _____

Evidence _____   Evidence _____

_____   _____

When you have finished with this step, proceed to the next step.

<u>Step 3. Sharing Problems and Formulating Solutions</u> (20 minutes)

Find two other teams of two so that you form groups of six. Go over your list of problems which you defined in the previous step for each of the grievances. Come to consensus as a group on what problems are reflected in each grievance. Write the list of problems on which your group agrees in the spaces provided below.

When you have agreed on the list of problems, then develop a suggested solution for each of the problems (i.e., what would you, as a consultant, suggest be done to help Brooksville State Hospital with each of these problems?).

CHUCK WHEELER'S GRIEVANCE　　　　　FORENSIC UNIT'S GRIEVANCE

Problem _____　　　Problem _____

_____　　　_____

Solution _____　　　Solution _____

_____　　　_____

Problem _____　　　Problem _____

_____　　　_____

Solution _____　　　Solution _____

_____　　　_____

Problem _____　　　Problem _____

_____　　　_____

Solution _____　　　Solution _____

_____　　　_____

When you have finished with this step, proceed to the next step.

Step 4. Evaluating Solutions (15 minutes)

Stay with the same group with which you worked in the prior step. Take each of the solutions you formulated in that step and evaluate them by each of the following criteria:

1. Did the suggested solution favor management or the employee?

2. Did the suggested solution contribute to better performance on the part of the immediate supervisor, or to better procedures for handling grievances on the part of the hospital?

3. Was the suggested solution short term or long range? That is, did it alleviate only the immediate problem, or did it set precedent for similar problems in the future?

Fill in the chart on the following page in order to answer each of these questions.

Complete the following chart with one- or two-word summations of each of your solutions from the prior step and then indicate in each of the boxes to which aspect of each criterion the solution speaks.

Solution	Management or Employee?	Supervisor or Hospital?	Short Term or Long Range?

CHUCK WHEELER

FORENSIC UNIT

Step 5. Debriefing (10 minutes)

1. Below is one set of "answers" to this frame, developed by the simulation designers. Working within your group of six, compare these "answers" to the ones you developed in the course of working through this frame. With which of these do you agree, and why? With which of these do you disagree, and why? (More questions on the following page!)

	Problem	Solution	Management or Employee?	Supervisor or Hospital?	Short Term or Long Range?
CHUCK WHEELER	Jackson's handling of Wheeler after filing of grievance	Stop therapy with Wheeler; order him to perform his duties correctly & attend staff meetings	management	supervisor	long range (Hopefully, her new behavior will carry over into other situations)
	Wheeler's attitude toward Jackson & level of work peformance	Remind Wheeler he's still probationary & can be refused permanent Civil Service status at end of 6 months if there is no improvement	management	hospital	short term
	Incongruence between interview & job assignment	Create written hospital policy re: promising job assignment during interviews	employee & management	hospital	long range
FORENSIC UNIT	Employees' disrupting staff meetings	Supervisor asks them not to bring up subject of grievance during staff meeting as it doesn't pertain to Social Services	management	supervisor	short term
	State's regulation on hazardous duty pay	Filing of grievance is itself a solution	employee	hospital	long range

2. Do you think that Chuck Wheeler's charge of racism is valid? (Remember that the two units vary in their racial composition by only 6%, and approximately 25% of the Social Services staff is black.)

3. Was Ms. Jackson's approach to Chuck Wheeler an example of good managerial practice, or good casework practice? Which do you think is more appropriate to a supervisor-employee situation such as the one in this scenario?

4. Did the majority of your group's solutions favor management or employees? Do you think this is appropriate for a supervisor?

5. To what extent is the Wheeler case racist in its presentation?

FRAME III

HANDLING GRIEVANCES IN A UNIONIZED SETTING

Step 1. Setting the Scene (5 minutes)

Western State Hospital is a large, state-owned institution in a fairly remote part of the state. Of its total population of 1,300, approximately 350 are geriatric. During its last session, the Legislature mandated deinstitutionalization for many of the state's wards. For Western State Hospital, this means that 300 of their 350 geriatric patients will be discharged from the hospital and placed in community-based facilities, both public and private, such as nursing homes, day care centers, and the like.

Western State Hospital is not alone in responding to the legislative mandate to deinstitutionalize many of its patients. Several states are following this route in an attempt to respond positively to charges that state institutions are no more than custodial warehouses for those persons with whom society doesn't wish to bother (such as the elderly, the mentally handicapped, and the emotionally disturbed). Deinstitutionalization means moving these persons from large, often physically isolated state institutions into smaller, community-based facilities. It is a movement that has grown concomitantly in the last 10 years with the drive for community mental health and the effort to guarantee the rights of mental patients to adequate treatment. If deinstitutionalization is successful through the use of high quality community-based facilities, then the individual patient can make significant progress in returning to independent living with treatment and support services tailored to the individual. If deinstitutionalization is not successful due to insufficient and/or inadequate community-based facilities, then the individual often is placed in a revolving-door situation in which the likelihood of return to the state hospital is greatly increased.

Western State Hospital has little control over community-based facilities in order to guarantee the kind of care that will be needed by their geriatric patients. Western State's program for the elderly is geared toward both maintenance and habilitation. Staff for this program includes: 94 psychiatric aides, 75 RNs, 25 LPNs, 5 social workers, 2 psychologists, 1 medical doctor, 2 occupational therapists, 2 recreational therapists, and 2 recreation aides. The psychiatric and recreation aides and the LPNs belong to a union, Local 841 American Federation of State, County, and Municipal Employees. The union steward of Local 841 AFSCME has filed a grievance with the superintendent of Western State Hospital over the future discharge of 300 of the hospital's 350 geriatric patients. This shift will take place within the next six months and threatens to eliminate many union jobs at the hospital. The grievance contends that the mass discharge of patients into community facilities is in direct violation of the first clause of the union's contract with Western State Hospital, "In order to provide the best possible patient care, this contract . . ." (Santiestevan, 1975).

According to the contract, the following steps must be taken to resolve a grievance:

STEP 1   FILING of original grievance by Grievants and
           Local Union Steward

STEP 2   HEARING: Grievants and Local Union Steward

STEP 3   DECISION by Hospital Superintendent

STEP 4   appeal

STEP 5   HEARING: Grievants and Local Union Steward "vs."
           Hospital Superintendent

STEP 6   DECISION by State Mental Health Program Director

STEP 7   appeal

STEP 8   HEARING: Grievants and State Union Steward "vs."
           Hospital Superintendent and State Mental Health
           Program Director

STEP 9   DECISION by State Civil Service Commission

STEP 10   appeal

STEP 11   HEARING: Grievants and State/National Union Steward "vs."
           Hospital Superintendent, State Mental Health Program
           Director, and other state officials

STEP 12   DECISION by the courts
           (final and binding; no appeal)

These time limits must be strictly adhered to:

> Ten (10) calendar days between filing of original grievance and first hearing

> Five (5) calendar days between conclusion of hearing and announcement of decision

> Five (5) calendar days between announcement of decision and filing of appeal

> Ten (10) calendar days between filing of appeal and next hearing

Step 2. Sorting Out the Evidence (20 minutes)

The fight between the hospital and the union has been going on for some time now. The union has lost all decisions and has appealed their grievance. The next hearing is to be held by the State Civil Service Commission. The duty of the Commission is to protect the rights of employees and of management (that is, the hospital administration and the state bureaucracy). In addition, the Commission is subject to political pressure: no state official connected with this grievance wants to see it go to final arbitration by the courts. The publicity surrounding the event and the possible decision could have adverse political effects on the state in this election year.

Likewise, the stewards in the union also feel political pressure. They are generally elected (sometimes appointed) and hence feel they must produce settlements favorable to the union if they are to retain their offices. Accordingly, they may sometimes take stands that are more radical than the majority of union members, or the "average" union member, would endorse.

In this step and in Step 3, you are a member of the State Civil Service Commission and you have 10 days in which to review the evidence. Remember that the union's grievance is essentially this:

> Transferring 300 of Western State Hospital's 350 geriatric patients to community facilities does not guarantee patients the continuation of proper care which they have been receiving at Western State. The burden is on management to demonstrate that the change will improve health care; to date, they have not done so. Indeed, evidence from other states (New York, Massachusetts, California) indicates that health care for the individual patient radically declines when the patient is moved from a state institution to a

community facility. Quality patient care is a key
feature of the Local 841 AFSCME contract. In
addition, wholesale transfer of patients from
Western State Hospital to community facilities does
not protect workers' job rights.

The hospital's counterargument is essentially this:

The decision to deinstitutionalize was made in the
legislature, not at Western State Hospital. The
union's contract is between the hospital and the
union, not between the legislature and the union.
Accordingly, Western State Hospital is implementing
a policy which was mandated by a body over which it
has no control. Quality care will, of course, continue
to be provided to patients left in Western State
Hospital's care. In addition, the contract clearly
states that layoffs and reduction in work forces are
not grievable--that is, they are not subject to
negotiation between union and the hospital except
during the time the contract is being renewed. The
contract is still in effect and, thus, the issue of
layoffs of union workers is not a legitimate basis
for grievance.

Your job is now to review the evidence submitted on behalf of each side
to see

--whether it speaks directly to the charge stipulated
  in the grievance;

--whether it is within the allowable time limits;

--whether it is official (that is signed, dated, etc.);

--whether it truly documents what it claims to document.

Individually, review each of the following pieces of evidence.
Write on the bottom of each document whether you, as a member of the
State Civil Service Commission, consider it to be valid or invalid and
why, for the purposes of the hearing you will be conducting.

When each participant has finished with this step, proceed to the
next step in this frame.

DOCUMENT #1

WESTERN STATE HOSPITAL

GRIEVANCE

Date: _January 1, 1976_

Name: _J. S. Gaffney_   *JS Gaffney*

Unit: _Geriatric Unit_

Grievance: _____ *transfer of hospital's geriatric patients to private facilities violates union contract, as this transfer "... does not provide best possible patient care ..." Transfer also does not protect workers' job rights.*

_____*JS Gaffney*_____
(Signed)

L.P.N. I, Geriatric Unit & Steward, Local AFSCME #841
(Rank)

_#76-1_   _January 15, 1976_

Grievance Number   Date

Disposition of Grievance: _Denied - transfer not in violation of contract; layoff of workers specifically non-grievable._

_____*A. P. Huntley*_____
(Signed)

DOCUMENT #2

January 3, 1976

M E M O R A N D U M

TO: Dr. H.P. Huntley, Superintendent,
          Western State Hospital

FROM: J.S. Gaffney, Steward, Local #841, AFSCME

SUBJECT: Documentation for Grievance #76-1

     Listed below are figures for states similar to ours which have
deinstitutionalized on a wholesale basis. The figures prove beyond
a doubt that quality care for citizens is greatly reduced after mass
deinstitutionalization is implemented. Other figures are included to
support this point.

   1. In 1975, there were 1.2 million long-term carebeds. At
      least 800,000 more are needed. Only 7% of the existing
   beds are approved by the Joint Commission on Accreditation
   of Hospitals.

   2. Of the nation's 23,000 nursing homes, more than half have
      had serious incidents of deliberate physical abuse or per-
   sonal injury to patients.

   3. Only 7,318 nursing homes are certified skilled nursing
      homes and more than half of these fail to meet fire safety
   requirements.

   4. In California, the population in the state's mental hos-
      pitals dropped 34,955 from 1963 to 1973. Hospitals for
   the mentally retarded declined 2,730 persons in the same period.

   5. In Massachussetts, all youthful offender institutions were
      closed and the crime rate went up.

JSG:ejd

DOCUMENT #3

January 5, 1976

M E M O R A N D U M

TO: Dr. H.P. Huntley, Superintendent,
        Western State Hospital

FROM: J.S. Gaffney, Steward, Local #841, AFSCME

SUBJECT: Grievance #76-1

    I have done some projections on what deinstitutionalization will
mean to the Geriatric Program. Under the state's current funding for-
mula, reducing the geriatric patient population from 350 to 50 will
mean the following staff will be left:

        14 psychiatric aides
        11 RN's
         1 LPN
        ½ social worker
        ¼ psychologist

    This leaves absolutely no medical doctor, or occupational or re-
creational therapists. Obviously, the treatment of geriatric patients
which has been such an integral part of this hospital will go down
the drain. This will ruin the quality of patient care for those few
remaining after the transfers have taken place.

    In addition, the job rights of 148 AFSCME members will be de-
nied. I would remind you that the average AFSCME member in the Geriatric Program has seniority of 3 years and 7 months. This is higher
than any other program at Western State.

JSG:ejd

DOCUMENT #4

January 25, 1976

<u>M E M O R A N D U M</u>

TO: Dr. J.T. Whiddon, Director
           State Mental Health Program

FROM: Dr. H.P. Huntley, Superintendent *H.P.H.*
           Western State Hospital

SUBJECT: Grievance #76-1

This memorandum serves to outline more fully to you the reasoning for denying Grievance #76-1. I am giving you this information for your consideration in hearing the appeal filed by the union, Local #841, AFSCME.

The union's first contention is that the quality of patient care will decline if the mass transfer to community facilities takes place. This simply is not true for the patients <u>remaining</u> at Western State Hospital. The staff-patient ratio will remain the same and, as you know, I have already made arrangements for rehabilitation efforts to be continued through other programs at Western State. In addition, Western State will assume some responsibility for the quality of care given to persons by other facilities after those persons are transferred from Western State. I shall assign two social workers to provide follow-up services.

The second contention by the union concerns the layoffs which will take place when the patient transfer takes place. This layoff will be necessitated by overwhelming budgetary considerations (i.e., the loss of 300 patients). Lay-offs due to budget reductions are solely the right of management and are not subject to grievance under the current contract (Section 9.41 of the contract).

JTW:ebs

DOCUMENT #5

February 11, 1976

MEMORANDUM

TO: A. Baxter, Director
        State Civil Service Commission

FROM: J.S. Gaffney, Steward   *J.S. Gaffney*
        Local Union #841, AFSCME

SUBJECT: Appeal of Grievance #76-1

This memorandum is to advise you that we are appealing the decision of Dr. H.P. Huntley, Superintendant of Western State Hospital concerning Grievance #76-1. Said decision was announced on February 4, 1976.

In addition to us, please notify V.R. Untermeyer, who is the State Steward of AFSCME, before the Commission.

JSG:ejd

DOCUMENT #6

February 17, 1976

M E M O R A N D U M

TO: Honorable Members of the State
           Civil Service Commission

FROM: V.R. Untermeyer,
           State Wide Steward, AFSCME

SUBJECT: Grievance #76-1, Western State Hospital

    I have personally reviewed the evidence presented by J.S. Gaffney
to Dr. H.P. Huntley prior to the original hearing. It is well
documented and accurate. I have personally checked all the facts and
can vouch for their accuracy. I believe they prove our point.

    I am taking this opportunity to inform you that identical
grievances to Grievance #76-1, Western State Hospital, are being filed
today at all AFSCME unionized state facilities which are undergoing
any form of deinstitutionalization.

VRU:jkg

Step 3. Sharing Responses (10 minutes)

    Participants should divide into groups of five, six, or seven in
order to compare their own evaluations of each of the documents in the
prior step. When they have come to a tentative conclusion as to their
validity and appropriateness, turn the page to compare your evaluations
with those of the simulation designers.

            Document #1 _____

            Document #2 _____

            Document #3 _____

            Document #4 _____

            Document #5 _____

            Document #6 _____

Evaluations of Documents in Step 2

Document #1 - Filing of original grievance and decision of first
    hearing. This document is perfectly acceptable.

Document #2 - Union's attempt to substantiate their grievance. These
    figures apply to places other than Western State Hospital. The
    union may use this data for background but they must also speak
    directly to conditions at Western State. Not acceptable as
    direct substantiation.

Document #3 - Union's attempt to substantiate their grievance. Unless
    the hospital can prove otherwise, the union is correct in its
    statement that the treatment of geriatric patients will be greatly
    reduced once the geriatric patient population drops to 50. Mass
    layoffs due to economic reasons (i.e., loss of 300 patients) is
    management's right and not subject to grievance. Therefore the
    second portion of the memorandum is not acceptable.

Document #4 - Superintendent's attempt to substantiate his decision
    against the union. He should have written proof (i.e., written
    agreement) concerning the continuation of habilitation once the
    patient population drops. This weakens but does not invalidate
    the claim. The second portion, concerning management's rights
    to lay off employees, is right on target.

Document #5 - Technically, this appeal was filed one day beyond the
    five-day limit for filing appeals. Accordingly, you could
    refuse to hear the appeal on the basis of a missed deadline.
    However, it is really up to Western State Hospital to bring
    this to your attention. Even if they do, tradition in labor
    grievance negotiations is that the deadlines to which grievants
    must adhere are somewhat flexible but deadlines for management
    are not. Also, from the hospital's point of view, they should
    probably prefer to deny the grievance on a more substantive
    basis than a technicality.

Document #6 - Memo from state union steward. This is a pressure
    tactic and a not-so-veiled threat. Has nothing to do with the
    actual grievance. Should be thrown out as evidence.

Step 4. The Hearing (15 minutes)

Now it is time for the State Civil Service Commission to hold its hearing on Grievance #76-1, Western State Hospital. Participants should stay in the same group which was formed in the last step. Your instructor will assign the following roles:

Superintendent, Western State Hospital;
Hospital's Legal Counsel;
Union's Legal Counsel;
Director of Civil Service Commission;
Observer #1;
Observer #2.

Each participant should turn to the role play instructions for his/her role on one of the following pages and read only that role. Do not read anyone else's role.

When each participant has read his/her role description, begin the role play. The director of the Commission will open the hearing and call on the superintendent to give testimony. Counsel for the hospital will have five (5) minutes to question the superintendent, as well as the counsel for the union. Remember that the procedures used loosely follow a court of law (that is, either counsel may object to testimony or questions, but nothing may be stricken from the record). No conclusions are to be reached in this role play; merely run the role play for ten (10) minutes.

Then proceed to the next step.

Role Play Instructions for <u>Superintendent</u>

You are a Ph.D. psychologist and have been Superintendent at Western State Hospital for two years. You take a great deal of pride in your program. You feel you have done a lot with few resources. You have tried to be as patient as you can with the union. But this last grievance is, in your personal opinion, totally ludicrous. For one thing, the hospital had no control over the legislature's mandate. You personally testified against it. You really don't like the union and see it as an intrusion upon your right to administer your program but accept the reality of its existence. Your denial of the grievance was based on two factors:

  --quality of care would remain the same after the
    transfer as before;

  --mass layoffs are a right of management and hence
    not grievable.

Review Documents 1 and 4 to refresh your memory.

Role Play Instructions for <u>Union's Legal Counsel</u>

The Superintendent has been extremely unresponsive to the unionized staff, in your opinion. You did not like the way she handled the original hearing. You also wish to challenge her on the basis that she has only two years experience in geriatrics. The local union steward has had 15 years of experience. You will challenge Document 4 on the basis that there is no proof about continuation of habilitation (i.e., a written agreement between Geriatrics and other programs at Western State).

Review Documents 1, 2, 3, 4, and 5 to refresh your memory.

Role Play Instructions for the <u>Hospital's Legal Counsel</u>

You wish to bring out two main points in your questioning of the Superintendent: (1) that quality of patient care will remain the same, regardless of transfers; and (2) management has a right to lay off employees and this right is, by definition, not grievable. You will want to discredit Documents 2 and 3. The information on patient care in other states is not relevant to Western State. Also, patient-staff ratios will remain the same. You will object to any efforts on the part of union's legal counsel to discredit the Superintendent or Document 4. Accordingly, you will challenge the union's legal counsel fairly often.

Review Documents 1, 2, 3, 4, and 5 to refresh your memory.

Role Play Instructions for <u>Director of the Commission</u>

Your main job is to listen carefully to each question and answer during this hearing. You are also to rule on objections made by either counsel, either to sustain them or to deny them. Be certain to allow each counsel only 5 minutes for questioning the superintendent.

Role Play Instructions for <u>Observers</u>

You are to watch the superintendent carefully and rate his/her performance as a witness according to the following model. At the end of the role play, you should have evaluated the superintendent on each of the items listed below (Patterson & Snyder, 1975).

	Strongly Agree	Agree	Do Not Know	Disagree	Strongly Disagree
1. Tells the truth	_____	_____	_____	_____	_____
2. Says he/she doesn't know when he/she doesn't	_____	_____	_____	_____	_____
3. Understands questions completely before answering	_____	_____	_____	_____	_____
4. Answers questions completely	_____	_____	_____	_____	_____
5. Doesn't volunteer information	_____	_____	_____	_____	_____
6. Quits talking if either counsel starts to speak	_____	_____	_____	_____	_____
7. Never explains or justifies answers	_____	_____	_____	_____	_____
8. Testimony spontaneous, not memorized	_____	_____	_____	_____	_____
9. Did not act angry, hostile, belligerent, sarcastic, etc.	_____	_____	_____	_____	_____
10. Did not let opposing counsel "get his/her goat"	_____	_____	_____	_____	_____
11. Did not hesitate to admit he/she didn't know something	_____	_____	_____	_____	_____

Step 5. Debriefing (10 minutes)

1. Stay in your small group. Have each observer share his/her evaluations of the superintendent with the group. Then ask the person who played the superintendent for his or her reactions.

2. Listed below are the four guidelines for sorting out good documentation from bad documentation. Also listed below are one person's ratings of the importance of each of these guidelines, with "1" being the most important and "4" being the least important. Do you agree with all these rankings? Why or why not? If you disagree, rank the items in what you feel is the appropriate order.

Another's Rank	Your Rank	Guideline
2	_____	Whether it speaks directly to the charge stipulated in the grievance
1	_____	Whether it is within the allowable time limits
3	_____	Whether it is official (that is, signed, dated, etc.)
4	_____	Whether it truly documents what it claims to document

REFERENCES

Patterson, L. T., & Snyder, F. B. The grievance handbook.
    Burlingame, Calif.: Association of California School
    Administrators, 1975.

Santiestevan, H. Deinstitutionalization: Out of their beds and into
    the streets. Washington, D. C.: American Federation of State,
    County, and Municipal Employees, 1975.

RELATED READINGS

Baer, W. E. Grievance handling: 101 guides for supervisors.
    New York: American Management Association, Inc., 1970.

Grievance guide. Washington, D. C.: Bureau of National Affairs,
    Inc., 1972.

Grievance procedures for teachers in negotiation agreements, Research
    Report 1969-R8. Washington, D. C.: National Education
    Association, 1969.

Lutz, F. W., Kleinman, L., & Evans, S. Grievances and their
    resolution. Danville, Ill.: The Interstate Printers and
    Publishers, Inc., 1967.

Scott, W. G. The management of conflict: Appeal systems in
    organizations. Homewood, Ill.: Richard D. Erwin, Inc., and the
    Dorsey Press, 1965.

Terry, G. R. Supervisor management. Homewood, Ill.: Richard D.
    Irwin, Inc., 1974.

Thomson, A. W. I. The grievance procedure in the private sector.
    Ithaca, N. Y.: New York State School of Industrial and Labor
    Relations, Cornell University, 1974.

MAXRAS: MAXIMIZING RESOURCES FOR AGENCY SURVIVAL

I. INTRODUCTION

In times of shrinking financial resources, human service organizations often have a difficult time obtaining needed funds to meet their objectives. Agency survival means more than just whether an agency exists; it also includes how well the agency is doing its work and what percentage of the target population it is reaching. One agency does not struggle for survival in a vacuum since it usually operates in a network of services. This network represents a pattern of interorganizational relationships (e.g., referral resources, funding resources, political resources, etc.) which play an important part in any one agency's survival.

In this simulation, participants will work with one very important aspect of interagency relationships--referring clients from one agency to another. Participants will work in one of five different agencies in the city of Huntington. All of these agencies are involved with children's mental health services, and they refer clients among one another.

II. GOAL AND ENABLING OBJECTIVES

Goal:

> To acquaint participants with the forces which impact
> on human service agencies and which influence the
> decision-making processes of those agencies.

Enabling Objectives:

1. Engage in case management.

2. Plan referral processes.

3. Engage in case coordination.

4. Maintain client-information systems.

5. Plan future service patterns based on service information.

III. PROCEDURES

FRAME I - Resource Assessment (20 minutes)

    Step 1. Service Capacity
    Step 2. Examination of Client Population

FRAME II - Intake and Referral (45 minutes)

    Step 1. Deciding Whom to Accept and Whom to Refer
    Step 2. Intake of New Clients
    Step 3. Negotiating Referrals
    Step 4. Recordkeeping
    Step 5. Evaluation

FRAME III - Client Treatment (30 minutes)

    Step 1. Recording Assignment of Clients to Service Units
    Step 2. Determining Treatment Success
    Step 3. Summarizing Treatment Success
    Step 4. Evaluating Treatment Success

FRAME IV - Resource Assessment and Program Planning (20 minutes)

    Step 1. Calculating Resources
    Step 2. Program Planning and Resource Allocation
    Step 3. Evaluating Resources and Planning

FRAME V - Second Round

    Step 1. Intake and Referrals (30 minutes)
    Step 2. Treatment (20 minutes)
    Step 3. Resource Allocation (10 minutes)

FRAME VI - Debriefing (20 minutes)

    Step 1. Agency Perspective
    Step 2. Participant Perspective

Materials Needed to Play MAXRAS

1. 3 x 5 index cards (for keeping track of clients).

2. 5 x 8 index cards (for agency identification place cards).

3. Notepads and pencils for agency recordkeeping.

4. "Success slips" in a cup, one cup for each team. The "success slips" are ten small pieces of paper of equal size with a different number--10%, 20%, 30%, 40%, 50%, 60%, 70%, 80%, 90%, and 100%.

INTRODUCTION TO MAXRAS

THE CITY OF HUNTINGTON AND ITS AGENCIES

Huntington is located in New England. It was founded prior to the Revolutionary War and has slowly grown from a farming village to a city of 185,000 which depends upon both light industry and the surrounding agricultural areas for its economic well-being. The nearest city of comparable size is 75 miles away. Nestled in the middle of the Berkshire Mountains, Huntington's human service agencies also serve the needs of the surrounding counties.

Five of these human service agencies are involved with children's mental health. They are state and local, public and private. They are:

AGENCY I: STATE HOSPITAL
Relatively few beds devoted to children's mental health. Mainly forced to accept children whom other agencies do not want. Would like to start innovative treatment programs but is unable to do so, due to nature of client population and relatively limited monetary and staff resources.

AGENCY II: COUNTY CHILD WELFARE
Part of the County Department of Public Welfare. Primarily a referral agency heavily loaded with a variety of child welfare problems including neglect, abuse, day care, adoptions, foster care, and children in need of supervision. Has limited resources and large caseloads. Limited in direct service capacity but must engage in case coordination processes in order to justify its cost effectiveness at budget preparation time each year.

AGENCY III: RESIDENTIAL TREATMENT CENTER
Private and local. Committed to traditional institutional care and does not have the expertise to handle changes in their approach to therapy. Dependent upon referrals from public agencies and private practitioners. Must plan its case coordination very closely (thereby minimizing the number of cases they refer to public institutions) in order to survive. Its inpatient and day-treatment caseload is the primary basis for securing financial resources.

AGENCY IV: COMMUNITY MENTAL HEALTH CENTER
               Focuses on day care for disturbed children,
               parent counseling, preventive mental health
               services in schools, and multidiscipline team
               approach to service provision. Sees the state
               hospital as the last resort; uses it primarily
               as place to which they transfer "unresponsive
               cases." Relies primarily on federal funding.
               Due to increases in county funds, must now
               engage in better case management strategies in
               order more effectively to coordinate with other
               local agencies.

AGENCY V: JUVENILE COURT
               Primarily a referral agency aimed at reducing its
               own caseload through extensive coordination with
               other agencies which can provide direct services.
               Has high volume of cases and is subject to local
               political pressure to refer "difficult kids" to
               state hospital. Gets assistance for cases from
               local public and private agencies but, for the
               most part, is dependent on the goodwill of these
               agencies to accept its referrals. Caught in a
               squeeze between a directive of the Juvenile Court
               judge to reduce caseloads and the increasing
               number of referrals from local law enforcement
               agencies. Thus, better case management strategies
               and better work relationships with local agencies
               for more direct services for children are needed.

PARTICIPATING IN MAXRAS

In this simulation each of you will be assigned to one agency.
You will serve as a staff member of the same agency throughout this
simulation. The simulation is divided into three basic parts:
Round 1 (Frames I through IV), Round 2 (Frame V), and Debriefing
(Frame VI). Round 1 represents one fiscal year in an agency's life.
After an entire year of referring and treating clients, agency staff
assess how it has done and then plan the service capacity for the next
year. Round 2 is the next fiscal year and is essentially the same as
Round 1. At the end of Round 2, agency staff again review the year to
see how they have done and plan for the third fiscal year. The staff
will also have a chance to compare their performances from one year
(Round 1) to the next (Round 2) and thus see how well or how poorly
their agency has survived.

In order to explain the details of this simulation, we shall now "walk through" the primary activities of Round 1. Each agency must first examine its capacity for service to clients and its client population. There are three different types of service an agency may offer and three different types of clients an agency may receive. In Frame II, each agency will decide which clients to accept from the new client population pool and which of its current clients to refer to other agencies based on its service capacity and plans for the future. Then the agencies will engage in the actual process of negotiating referrals with other agencies. In Frame III, clients within each agency will be treated by a "chance" draw of a number, and the success or failure of treatment will be recorded. In Frame IV, each agency will assess its resources in light of the number of clients it had and how successfully it treated each client. Based upon the completed resource assessment, an agency will plan its program for the next year (Round 2).

The entire simulation involves a certain amount of risk taking. If an agency is to keep its status quo or enhance it, it must gamble by taking on more clients than it has service capacity. It must also gamble in assigning its clients to one of its three types of service units for treatment; it must decide if it wishes to overload one unit severely or overload each unit mildly. The outcome of these decisions will either pay off or harm the agency in resource assessment, for in each round your agency will be:

--rewarded for treating clients successfully;

--penalized for underutilizing your service capacity;

--penalized for failure to treat clients successfully.

In completing this simulation, agency staff should strike a balance between being excessively cautious and throwing reason to the wind. A reasoned chance is usually a good bet, and a bit of a gamble can pay off.

UNDERSTANDING THE THEORETICAL FOUNDATION FOR MAXRAS

The agencies of Huntington form a system among themselves. The agencies within this system operate in a network of interorganizational relationships. The one concept that most characterizes their relationships is exchange. In this simulation, the agencies in Huntington exchange clients among one another. As no one agency has everything it needs to survive, they exchange among themselves to get what they need to survive. This exchanging is voluntary in nature. They exchange primarily three elements: cases, staff, and other resources (such as equipment, technology, etc.). This simulation focuses only on case exchange. The amount of exchanging by any one agency depends upon three factors:

  --the accessibility of each organization to the clients not receiving its services;

  --the objectives of the organization and how resources are allocated to meet those objectives;

  --the degree to which the organizations within the system agree that each agency has a special contribution to make and that there is respect for the domain of each agency.

Of these three factors, the last factor, that of domain consensus, is important. An agency does not set its objectives in a vacuum. Rather, it decides what it will or will not do by considering what other agencies are doing in the same area and how likely those other agencies are to agree that one agency can do what it says it wants to do.

There are four main dimensions in the concept of exchange (Levine & White, 1974). The first is the parties to the exchange (e.g., agencies). The second is the type of exchange (e.g., regular or infrequent, appropriate or inappropriate cases, large or small amounts of information, etc.). The third is the agreement underlying the exchange (written or verbal, formal or informal, rigid or flexible, etc.). The fourth is the direction of the exchange (unilateral, reciprocal, or joint).

FRAME I

RESOURCE ASSESSMENT

Among all the simulation participants, count off from 1 to 5.
Each person with the number 1 will be Agency I; each person with the
number 2 will be Agency II; etc. You will remain as a staff member of
that agency for the entire simulation.

Take no more than 20 minutes to complete this frame.

Step 1. Service Capacity

Each agency team must now examine its capacity for service as
shown below. Each agency has a varying capacity of service units. One
service unit is capable of treating one client at an optimum level.

Since all forms of treatment cannot be included in this
simulation, three general types of treatment are shown below
(inpatient, outpatient, and day treatment). It can be seen that each
agency, depending on its purpose and role, has varying capacities at
the present time for inpatient, outpatient, and day treatment services
and usually refers clients whom they cannot serve to other agencies.
It must be remembered that "service unit capacity" refers to the number
of services an agency has available to clients. These services
represent capability to deliver "direct services" to clients. Each
service unit optimally serves one client. If more than one client is
added to a service unit, the quality of that service is severely
reduced and each additional client beyond the first client has a
reduced chance of successful treatment. As we can see in Table 1, the
state hospital has the largest capacity to deliver services in all
categories. The only other agency capable of delivering in all three
categories is the local community mental health center. While carrying
out the exercise, thought should be given to future plans related to
adding or subtracting services within your agency.

Table 1.   CAPACITY FOR SERVICE TO CLIENTS

AGENCY	Inpatient*	Day Treatment**	Outpatient***
I. State Hospital	13	2	1
II. County Child Welfare	0	0	6
III. Residential Treatment Center	6	2	0
IV. Community Mental Health Center	1	10	6
V. Juvenile Court	0	0	4

   *Inpatient: Child removed from home to institution and all treatment takes place in the institution.

   **Day Treatment: Child remains in the home but receives day care treatment within the agency.

   ***Outpatient: Child remains in the home and receives outpatient treatment, while parents receive family therapy.

Step 2.   Examination of Client Population

   The following is a description of the client population served. There are three broad categories of client population:

   Client Type A - Severely emotionally disturbed children, or children with no home (deceased parents). There are only a few of these clients (5%).

   Client Type B - Severe pathology in the home affecting either child, parent, or both. These cases are resistant to treatment and correction and represent 30% of the client population.

   Client Type C - Family structure under stress but viable. Agency treatment of the child is more beneficial when the family as a whole is treated. These children comprise 65% of clients.

Client A can be treated best on an inpatient basis. Client B can be treated best on a day treatment basis. Client C can be treated best on an outpatient basis. Table 2 gives the types and numbers of clients assigned initially to your agency.

Table 2. INITIAL ASSIGNMENT OF CLIENTS TO AGENCIES

	AGENCY	Client A	Client B	Client C
I.	State Hospital	1	3	10
II.	County Child Welfare	5	1	5
III.	Residential Treatment Center	1	3	2
IV.	Community Mental Health Center	1	3	5
V.	Juvenile Court	5	1	2

Now, fill out the chart below with the figures that apply to your agency.

	Number of Service Units	x	Capacity of Each Service Unit	=	Agency's Client Capacity	Agency's Assignment of Clients
Inpatient	_____	x	1	=	_____	_____ Client Type A
Day Treatment	_____	x	1	=	_____	_____ Client Type B
Outpatient	_____	x	1	=	_____	_____ Client Type C

This will allow you to compare your agency's capacity for serving clients with the number of clients initially assigned to your agency.

Now, make a separate index card to represent each client. Make one card for each client. Put "A" on the card for client type A, "B" for client type B, etc. This will serve to remind you exactly how many of each type of client you have in your agency.

FRAME II

INTAKE AND REFERRAL

When working through this frame, take no more than 40 minutes to complete the intake and referral process of Steps 1 through 4. You will need at least 5 minutes to answer the questions in Step 5.

Your analysis of your agency should have led to the realization that capacity to serve is not always matched neatly with the number and/or types of clients currently served by the agency. In order to work at full capacity, therefore, an agency often has to select new clients to "match" its service provision structure. This "match" is especially important since funding for next year will be based on the total number of clients served, given the agency's service capacity.

Remember that all agencies can expect to receive clients from other agencies (via referral) all through the year and each agency will, no doubt, refer clients whom it cannot serve. Remember, also, that your agency should not allow itself to lose service capacity in the future simply because your current caseload is light. In fact, for even those clients who fail in treatment, there may be success in using additional treatment before the client is referred out of your agency. If, of course, your agency has no capacity to serve a particular type of client (see Table 1), then the case must be referred. "Capacity building," or adding on agency service capacities, comes later in the simulation.

There are two types of information you will need to complete this step. They are as follows: (1) "new client population" available for acceptance by each agency; and (2) the rules for interagency referrals.

New Client Population. New clients are currently available for acceptance/intake by each agency. By type, they are as follows:

        Client Type A - one (1);
        Client Type B - four (4);
        Client Type C - eight (8).

Rules for Interagency Referrals. In making referrals to other agencies, the following ground rules apply:

1. Any agency may refuse a referral but must state reason to agency seeking to make referral;

2. Any agency seeking to refer a client must state reason for making request;

3. Any agency may refer to state hospital without negotiation;

4. Any agency except state hospital can refuse to accept a referral;

5. Any client not accepted by another agency must stay in the agency which initially attempted to refer that client.

In addition, each of you should now study Table 3 to determine which agencies can make and receive referrals.

Table 3.   ALLOWABLE REFERRAL TARGETS

State Hospital may refer only to Residential Treatment Center

County Child Welfare may refer to State Hospital, Community Mental Health Center, and Juvenile Court

Residential Treatment Center may refer only to State Hospital

Community Mental Health Center may refer to State Hospital and County Child Welfare

Juvenile Court may refer to State Hospital, Residential Treatment Center, and Community Mental Health Center

---

Step 1. Deciding Whom to Accept and Whom to Refer

Using Tables 1, 2, and 3, noted again on the next page for your convenience, each agency should determine the types of clients which it is best prepared to serve (i.e., review your service capacity to see what types of services you can now offer). Also, review the number and types of clients you currently have in relation to your service capacity. This information is on the chart you completed in the first frame.

Table 1. CAPACITY FOR SERVICE TO CLIENTS

AGENCY	Inpatient*	Day Treatment**	Outpatient***
I. State Hospital	13	2	1
II. County Child Welfare	0	0	6
III. Residential Treatment Center	6	2	0
IV. Community Mental Health Center	1	10	6
V. Juvenile Court	0	0	4

*Inpatient: Child removed from home to institution and all treatment takes place in the institution.

**Day Treatment: Child remains in the home but receives day care treatment within the agency.

***Outpatient: Child remains in the home and receives outpatient treatment, while parents receive family therapy.

Table 2. INITIAL ASSIGNMENT OF CLIENTS TO AGENCIES

AGENCY	Client A	Client B	Client C
I. State Hospital	1	3	10
II. County Child Welfare	5	1	5
III. Residential Treatment Center	1	3	2
IV. Community Mental Health Center	1	3	5
V. Juvenile Court	5	1	2

Table 3. ALLOWABLE REFERRAL TARGETS

State Hospital may refer only to Residential Treatment Center

County Child Welfare may refer to State Hospital, Community Mental Health Center, and Juvenile Court

Residential Treatment Center may refer only to State Hospital

Community Mental Health Center may refer to State Hospital and County Child Welfare

Juvenile Court may refer to State Hospital, Residential Treatment Center, and Community Mental Health Center

Then, do the following:

1. Decide how many (if any) and what types of clients you are willing to accept--both from the "new client population" and by means of referral from other agencies. Also, decide which type(s) and how many of your current clients you would like to refer to other agencies.

2. Keep a record of your decisions at the top of the next page on the form "Intake and Referral." Under Section I, "Intake," note why you want certain types of new clients and how many of each type. Under Section II, "Referrals," note why you wish to refer certain types of clients and how many of each. Also, note to which agency you would like to refer each one.

INTAKE AND REFERRAL

I. INTAKE

Number of
Clients Desired   Reasons

Type A   _____   _____

                     _____

                     _____

Type B   _____   _____

                     _____

                     _____

Type C   _____   _____

                     _____

                     _____

II. REFERRAL

Number of Clients to Be Referred	Reasons	Agency to Which Clients Should Be Referred
Type A _____	_____	_____
	_____	_____
	_____	_____
Type B _____	_____	_____
	_____	_____
	_____	_____
Type C _____	_____	_____
	_____	_____
	_____	_____

Step 2. Intake of New Clients

Accept as many new clients from the "new client population" pool, up to the maximum number allowed per type as listed in the first part of this frame. Remember to leave yourself some negotiating room. That is, although it is desirable to have all your service units filled, you may need to trade off clients with another agency in order to refer a client you wish to get rid of.

To accept a new client, simply create a new index card for each new client. (For example, on a blank card, simply write the letter which represents the type of client--A, B, or C.)

New Client Population Available to Each Agency

   Client Type A - one (1)
   Client Type B - four (4)
   Client Type C - eight (8)

Step 3. Negotiating Referrals

Negotiate your referrals with the other four agencies. Remember to give a reason why you wish to send each referral. Refer to Table 3 and the rules preceding it for guidelines.

Step 4. Recordkeeping

After all referrals have been sent and received, tally the total number of clients which you currently have in each category (A, B, or C). This is your new caseload and these are the clients whom you will "treat" in the next frame.

   Number of Type A clients _____
   Number of Type B clients _____
   Number of Type C clients _____

Step 5. Evaluation

You have just completed a simulated exercise in intake and referral. On the basis of your experience, discuss the following questions:

1. Did the actions that took place reflect the agencies' interests, the clients' interests, or the interests of both? Explain.

2. Did any agency employ any "strategy" in its actions? For what purpose(s)?

3. Who, if anyone, played client advocate?

4. Was there a tendency to "dump" unwanted or hopeless cases on the state hospital? Was that anyone's concern?

FRAME III

CLIENT TREATMENT

Take no more than 25 minutes to complete client treatment
(Steps 1 through 3). You will need at least 5 minutes to answer the
questions in Step 4.

It is now time to provide treatment for your current caseload of
clients. A good treatment is one that is most appropriate for the
problem. For example, a Client A child with severe disturbance will
have a greater chance of success if removed from the home, while
conversely, there is less chance for success with a Client C child who
is placed in an institution.

Based on this rationale, success probabilities have been
established in Table 4 for each combination of type of case and type
of treatment.

Table 4. PROBABILITIES OF SUCCESS IN TREATMENT:
TYPE OF CASE BY TYPE OF TREATMENT

Type of Treatment	Type of Case		
	Client A	Client B	Client C
Inpatient	60%	30%	10%
Day Treatment	0%	50%	20%
Outpatient	0%	20%	60%

Based on the cases in your current caseload, it is now time to
match up "treatments" to "clients." It should be remembered that an
optimal caseload is one client per service unit. If your number and
types of service units are limited, you may choose to assign more than
one client per unit. Note, however, that when you do this, the second
client assigned to a unit has its probability of success (as listed in
Table 4) reduced by 10%; the third client has its probability of
success reduced by 20%, etc. You should decide if you wish to overload
all your service units equally or if you want to strain just one unit
but strain it to its utmost. Once a client is assigned to a unit, he/
she may not be switched to another unit.

Step 1. Recording Assignment of Clients to Service Units

This step involves agency case recordkeeping and general paperwork. Be very careful to keep accurate records; the state is planning to do a case-record audit on a state-wide basis in the very near future and your agency will not want to be caught short.

The directions for using Case Record Form T on the next page are as follows:

1. In Column 1, list each service unit for your agency once. For inpatient units, write IP on the line; for day treatment units, write DT; for outpatient units, write OP (see example in first two unnumbered lines of Form T). The total number of lines completed should match your agency's current number of service units (e.g., if you have two (2) inpatient units and seven (7) day treatment units, complete lines 1 through 9 (Column 1 only).

2. In Column 2 of Form T, match the clients in your current caseload with an appropriate service unit (see examples at top of Form T). If you have more clients than you have service units, you may need to overload your units. Overload cases (and their treatment success) can be noted in parentheses alongside the first case served in each unit (see example lines in Form T for clients A3 and A4). All your agency's clients must be assigned to a service unit.

RECORD FORM T

Type of Service Unit (Col. 1)	Client Type (Col. 2)	1st	2nd	3rd	4th	5th
EX: IP	A1 (A3)	S (F)	(S)			
IP	A2 (A4)	F (S)	F	S		
1.						
2.						
3.						
4.						
5.						
6.						
7.						
8.						
9.						
10.						
11.						
12.						
13.						
14.						
15.						
16.						
17.						
18.						
19.						
20.						
21.						
22.						
23.						

Step 2. Determining Treatment Success

In order to determine the success of treatment for each client in your caseload, it is necessary to draw one slip of paper from your cup of success slips for each client treatment. Compare the number on the slip with the probability of success figure listed for that type of client matched with that type of treatment in Table 4. If the number on the slip is equal to or lower than the probability of success, the treatment was a SUCCESS. If the number on the slip is higher than the probability of success, the treatment was a FAILURE.

If a client succeeds in the first treatment, record an "S" in the first column of Form T next to client. If the client fails, record an "F." Remember that the probability of success is reduced by 10% each time a client is treated (e.g., if client A in IP had a 60% probability of success, that probability is reduced to 50% for the next draw).

If there is very little or no chance for success by further treatment within one round, the case can be carried over to the next round but must carry the failure record. Keep drawing slips and recording failures for each client until that client succeeds or until five slips have been drawn for that client.

Remember: After each treatment (each draw), place the slips back into the cup and shake well before the next treatment.

Step 3. Summarizing Treatment Success

Each agency should prepare a brief summary of its recent treatment success by using the following chart. Simply total up the correct numbers from Record Form T.

SUMMARY OF TREATMENT SUCCESS, ROUND 1

Type of Client	Treated Successfully	Failed to Treat Successfully	Totals
A	_____	_____	_____
B	_____	_____	_____
C	_____	_____	_____
Totals =	_____	_____	_____

Step 4. Evaluating Treatment Success

Having completed a simulation exercise in treatment determination, discuss the following issues:

1. Were the opportunities for maximum success in treatment fully utilized?

2. What "value" decisions had to be made? Did these conflict with your own values?

3. Do you think that the probabilities of success in Table 4 are unrealistic? Why? How much <u>does</u> chance enter into the "real world" vis-a-vis success in treating people with mental problems? Do you believe in the old adage that of all clients served 1/3 get better, 1/3 get worse, 1/3 stay the same?

FRAME IV

RESOURCE ASSESSMENT AND PROGRAM PLANNING

When working through this frame, take no more than 15 minutes to complete Steps 1 and 2. Allow at least 5 minutes to answer the questions in Step 3.

Now that you have completed one round of play--which is to be considered as one year of your agency's operation--it is time to evaluate the characteristics of your current client caseload as related to your present ability to provide services (i.e., the number and types of service units which your agency now has). Further, it is time to review the number of resources--defined as energy + time + money--which your agency has, so that plans for the future can be made.

Step 1. Calculating Resources

Complete Form X for your agency. Parts 1, 2, and 3 reflect the resources which your agency has gained and/or lost during the past year as a result of its service provision activities. To assist you in completing Form X, four examples are given below.

Example 1.	Type of Client	# Successfully Treated	Resource Weight		
	A	1	.75	=	.75
	B	1	.50	=	.50
	C	3	.10	=	.30
			Gain Subtotal:		1.55

Example 2. If you treated 15 cases and you have only 7 <u>service units</u> (e.g., 1 IP, 3 DT, and 4 OP), then you should subtract 7 from 15 and you will have served 8 <u>excess cases</u>. This means you will receive 9 new resources.

Gain Subtotal: 9.00

Note: If your agency treated fewer cases than it had service units, you get <u>no</u> bonus resources here.

Excess Clients		Bonus Resources
1-2	leads to	2
3-6	leads to	5
7 or more	leads to	9

Example 3. Loss due to underutilization of service units.

Type of Service Units	# Began With	-	# Used	Difference	x	Wt.		
Inpatient	3	-	2	1	x	5	=	5.0
Day Treatment	1	-	1	0	x	2	=	0.0
Outpatient	2	-	2	0	x	1	=	0.0

Loss Subtotal: 5.0

Note: If your agency used 100% of its units, there is no loss of resources.

Example 4. If your agency started out with 20 resources (as Agency 4 did), and you gained 1.55 (for successful treatment) and 9.00 (for large numbers served), but lost 5.0 for underuse of your service program, your total number of resources would now be: 25.55.

FORM X: RESOURCES AVAILABLE

1. NEW RESOURCES GAINED FROM SUCCESSFUL TREATMENT OF CLIENTS

Type of Client	Number Successfully Treated	X	Resource Weight	=	Gain
A	_____	X	.75	=	_____
B	_____	X	.50	=	_____
C	_____	X	.10	=	_____
			GAIN SUBTOTAL:	+	_____

2. NEW RESOURCES GAINED FROM NUMBER OF CLIENTS SERVED

Note: If your agency treated fewer clients than it had client capacity, you get no bonus resources here.

Total number of cases served (regardless of success)   _____

MINUS Total number of service units (all three types)   - _____

EQUALS Number of excess clients served   _____

Excess Clients		Bonus Resources
1-2	leads to	2
3-6	leads to	5
7 or more	leads to	9

GAIN SUBTOTAL: + _____

3. LOSS OF RESOURCES DUE TO FAILURE TO USE ALL SERVICE UNITS

Note: If your agency used 100% of its units, there is no loss of resources here.

Type of Service Unit	Number Began With	-	Number Used	=	Difference	X	Weight	=	Loss
Inpatient	_____	-	_____	=	_____	X	5	=	_____
Day Treatment	_____	-	_____	=	_____	X	2	=	_____
Outpatient	_____	-	_____	=	_____	X	1	=	_____
							LOSS SUBTOTAL:	-	_____

4. LOSS OF RESOURCES DUE TO UNSUCCESSFUL TREATMENT OF CLIENTS

Type of Client	Number of Clients Unsuccessfully Treated	X	Resource Weight	=	Loss
A	_____	X	.75	=	_____
B	_____	X	.50	=	_____
C	_____	X	.10	=	_____
			LOSS SUBTOTAL:		−_____

5. NUMBER OF RESOURCES WITH WHICH YOUR AGENCY BEGAN ROUND 2

Copy the number listed below for your agency:

State Hospital	70
County Child Welfare	1
Private Residential Center	34
Community Mental Health Center	20
Juvenile Court	1

GAIN SUBTOTAL: +_____

6. GRAND TOTAL OF CURRENT RESOURCES

Subtotal from 1   _____

PLUS subtotal from 2   _____

PLUS subtotal from 5   +_____

    EQUALS   _____

MINUS subtotal from 3   −_____

    EQUALS   _____

MINUS subtotal from 4   −_____

    EQUALS   _____ GRAND TOTAL RESOURCES

Step 2. Program Planning and Resource Allocation

It is now time to plan for next year. You do not know how many referrals you will receive or what types of clients. Also, you have no idea how many (or what type of) new clients will be available from the "new client population." Thus, you must do the best you can in projecting the types and quantity of service units which you will need in the new year.

Remember that if you want to add, change, or relinquish service units, you may do so--but usually at a cost of resources (see Table 5 on the next page). For example, if you are the state hospital and you wish to drop one day treatment unit (as shown in Table 5, worth 4 resources) and to add one outpatient unit (which is worth 6 resources), this will cost 10 of your resources. A similar swap would cost county child welfare 14 resources, private residential center 16 resources, community mental health center 4 resources, and juvenile court no resources. Or the state hospital could simply add an outpatient unit at a cost of only 6 resources, etc.

A. Based on the resources that you currently have (the Grand Total Resources from Form X), devise a plan for service provision for the new year. What kinds of service units will you need? How many of each type? (Note: you can plan only within the limits allowed by your current quantity of resources). On the page entitled, "Program Plan and Resource Allocation," note any changes in service units which you would like to make. Also, note the cost in resources which each change would entail.

B. Justify your plan for service unit changes and use of your current resources. List your primary reasons for suggesting the changes you proposed in A above.

C. Take your "Plan" and justification to your instructor so it can be reviewed by an "outsider." If the instructor approves, you can assume that your desired changes will be put into effect before the new year begins.

Table 5.   RESOURCE COST TO ADD OR CHANGE SERVICE
CAPACITY (PER UNIT) FOR EACH AGENCY*

	AGENCY	Inpatient	Day Treatment	Outpatient
I.	State Hospital	2	4	6
II.	County Child Welfare	10	10	4
III.	Private Residential Center	2	6	10
IV.	Community Mental Health Center	10	2	2
V.	Juvenile Court	0	0	0

*Capacity type must be changed unit-for-unit. The total cost
of change is the sum of both units affected.

Note: Keep a paper record of your resources, since no tokens or forms
of recordkeeping are provided. Resources are defined here to
include MONEY + TIME + ENERGY, not simply money alone. For
example, it is difficult for a social service agency, like any
other organization, to change and any change requires the
expenditure of resources. Therefore, the cost of changing an
agency's ability to provide certain types of services is not
only a money cost but also a time and psychic energy cost to
the agency, all measured--in this exercise--in terms of
resources.

PROGRAM PLAN AND RESOURCE ALLOCATION

	SERVICE CAPACITY			RESOURCES
	Inpatient	Day Treatment	Outpatient	
Add	_____	_____	_____	_____
Delete	_____	_____	_____	_____
	_____	_____	_____ TOTAL	_____

A. Justification for addition of service capacity:

_____

_____

_____

_____

_____

_____

B. Justification for reduction of service capacity:

_____

_____

_____

_____

_____

_____

Step 3. Evaluating Resources and Planning

The resource allocation phase of this exercise offers a number of questions for discussion:

1. In reaching decisions about service unit changes, what values were expressed? Whose interests did they reflect?

2. What does funding on a per capita (or head-count) basis do to the quality of services which an agency is able to offer?

3. Should an agency "do what it has to" to survive? Or, if it cannot get sufficient funds to provide the services it deems appropriate, should it refuse to "play the game" and just go out of existence?

4. How realistic is it that changes in service units are quite costly to mental health agencies such as the ones simulated here?

FRAME V

SECOND ROUND

Round 2 proceeds in the same order as Round 1. First, put aside all client cards except those whom you treated unsuccessfully. The steps of play are as follows:

Step 1. Intake and Referrals (30 minutes)

A. Each agency examines its capacity for service. The number of clients per service unit which will yield optimum treatment has changed. Fill out the following chart for your agency:

Type of Unit	Number of Service Units*	x	Capacity of Each Unit	=	Agency's Client Capacity
Inpatient	_____	x	1	=	_____
Day Treatment	_____	x	2	=	_____
Outpatient	_____	x	3	=	_____
TOTAL CLIENT CAPACITY (IP + DT + OP)	_____				

*Copy these numbers from your "Program Plan and Resource Allocation" in the preceding frame.

B. Now, record the number of failures (the number of clients who are still in your agency) from the previous round.

Give half of these failures to the juvenile court (e.g., if there are 5, round to the higher number and send 3). Represent the failures with an "F" on the index card and then swap cards from the prior round to represent these clients.

		To/Received by Juvenile Court		Total Number of Clients in Agency
Type A _____	+	_____	=	_____
Type B _____	+	_____	=	_____
Type C _____	+	_____	=	_____

C. New Client Population - For each agency except county child welfare. The population is as follows:

Client Type	Number
A	2
B	10
C	20

The county child welfare must take at least one Type A client, three Type B clients, and five Type C clients.

D. Intake - Given the constraints of the clients who are failures from the prior round (and the number of new clients the county child welfare must take) decide how many new clients you wish to select; any clients not served may be returned to the state hospital at any time. Create new cards to represent each of your intakes. Fill out the "Intake and Referral" form on the following page.

E. Referral - Decide which of your clients you would like to refer to other agencies. Keep in mind the rules listed in Frame 1 for referrals. Complete the second half of the "Intake and Referral" form on the following page.

F. Negotiate your proposed referrals with other agencies. Once the referrals are negotiated, swap index cards to represent your new intakes.

G. After all referrals have been completed, tally the total number of each type of client:

Type A _____

Type B _____

Type C _____

INTAKE AND REFERRAL

I. INTAKE

Number of
Clients Desired   Reasons

Type A _____   _____

                    _____

                    _____

Type B _____   _____

                    _____

                    _____

Type C _____   _____

                    _____

                    _____

II. REFERRAL

Number of Clients to Be Referred	Reasons	Agency to Which Clients Should Be Referred
Type A _____	_____	_____
	_____	_____
	_____	_____
Type B _____	_____	_____
	_____	_____
	_____	_____
Type C _____	_____	_____
	_____	_____
	_____	_____

Step 2. Treatment (20 minutes)

    A.   Recall the probabilities of success of each combination of
client by type of treatment:

Table 4.   PROBABILITIES OF SUCCESS IN TREATMENT

Type of Treatment	Type of Case		
	Client A	Client B	Client C
Inpatient	60%	30%	10%
Day Treatment	0%	50%	20%
Outpatient	0%	20%	60%

    B.   Match treatments to clients. Remember that the optimal
caseloads per type of treatment have changed. Fill out
the first two columns of Record Form T (following page).
Circle those clients on the form who are failures, held
over from the first round.

    C.   You may switch clients from unit to unit. However, a
penalty of 10% (because a treatment failed) against the
probability of success will be levied on that client.

    D.   Begin to draw slips from the cup to treat your clients.
Remember that if the number drawn is equal to or lower
than the probability of success, the treatment was a
SUCCESS. If the number drawn is higher than the
probability of success, the treatment was a FAILURE.
Also remember to replace the slip after each draw and
shake the cup well before drawing again. The following
constraints apply:

        1.   Failures from the prior round (those clients
circled on Record Form T) begin with a 10%
lower probability of success than listed in
Table 4.

        2.   If a client is switched to another unit, he/she
is listed as a client under that unit, but the
probability of success has been reduced by 10%
(because it is not the initial treatment) and
the result is recorded under the appropriate
treatment schedule number.

        3.   If a FAILED client is transferred to a new unit
and that unit is already working at capacity,
then the probability of success is further
reduced by another 10%.

4. If a FAILED client remains in the same unit for treatment but that unit is already working at capacity, the probability of success is <u>further reduced by another 10%</u>.

E. Summarize your agency's treatment by totaling the correct numbers from Record Form T.

SUMMARY OF TREATMENT SUCCESS, ROUND 2

Type of Clients	Treated Successfully	Failed to Treat Successfully	Totals
A	_____	_____	_____
B	_____	_____	_____
C	_____	_____	_____

RECORD FORM T

Type of Service Unit (Col. 1)	Client Type (Col. 2)	1st	2nd	3rd	4th	5th
EX: IP	A1 (A3)	S (F)	(S)			
IP	A2 (A4)	F (S)	F	S		
1.						
2.						
3.						
4.						
5.						
6.						
7.						
8.						
9.						
10.						
11.						
12.						
13.						
14.						
15.						
16.						
17.						
18.						
19.						
20.						
21.						
22.						
23.						

Step 3. Resource Allocation (10 minutes)

A. Complete Form X, which appears below.

FORM X: RESOURCES AVAILABLE

1. NEW RESOURCES GAINED FROM SUCCESSFUL TREATMENT OF CLIENTS

Type of Client	Number Successfully Treated	X	Resource Weight	=	Gain
A	_____	X	.75	=	_____
B	_____	X	.50	=	_____
C	_____	X	.10	=	_____

GAIN SUBTOTAL: +_____

2. NEW RESOURCES GAINED FROM NUMBER OF CLIENTS SERVED

Note: If your agency treated fewer clients than it had client capacity, you get no bonus resources here.

Total number of cases served (regardless of success)   _____

MINUS Total number of service units (all three types)

	Service Capacity*		Capacity		Total Number
Inpatient	_____	X	1	=	_____
Day Treatment	_____	X	2	=	_____
Outpatient	_____	X	3	=	_____

*Obtain Service Capacity figure
from your "Program Plan and Resource
Allocation" in Frame IV, Step 2.

Total number of service units   -_____

EQUALS Number of excess clients served   =_____

GAIN SUBTOTAL: +_____

3. LOSS OF RESOURCES DUE TO FAILURE TO USE ALL CLIENT CAPACITY

   Note: If your agency used 100% of its units,
   there is no loss of resources.

Type of Service Unit	Number Began With	-	Number Used	=	Difference	X	Weight	=	Loss
Inpatient	_____	-	_____	=	_____	X	5	=	_____
Day Treatment	_____	-	_____	=	_____	X	2	=	_____
Outpatient	_____	-	_____	=	_____	X	1	=	_____
							LOSS SUBTOTAL:	-	_____

4. LOSS OF RESOURCES DUE TO UNSUCCESSFUL TREATMENT OF CLIENTS

Type of Client	Number of Clients Unsuccessfully Treated	X	Weight	=	Loss
A	_____	X	.75	=	_____
B	_____	X	.50	=	_____
C	_____	X	.10	=	_____
			LOSS SUBTOTAL:	-	_____

5. NUMBER OF RESOURCES WITH WHICH YOUR AGENCY BEGAN ROUND 2

   Copy this number from your "Program Plan and Resource
   Allocation" in Frame IV, Step 2.

                                          GAIN SUBTOTAL: + _____

6. GRAND TOTAL OF RESOURCES AT COMPLETION OF ROUND 2

        Subtotal from 1   _____

        PLUS subtotal from 2   _____

        PLUS subtotal from 5   +_____

           EQUALS   _____

        MINUS subtotal from 3   -_____

           EQUALS   _____

        MINUS subtotal from 4   -_____

           EQUALS   _____ GRAND TOTAL RESOURCES

    B. Compare your resources at three different points in time.

        --at the beginning of Round 1
          (see Form X in Frame IV)   _____

        --at the end of Round 1
          (see Form X in Frame IV)   _____

        --at the end of Round 2   _____

If your resources stayed the same or increased, then you can consider
your agency a success. If your resources decreased, then you can
consider your agency to be in trouble. Remember, however, that success
is relative. Some agencies may have been so handicapped from the first
that survival itself was a miracle.

FRAME VI

DEBRIEFING

Take 20 minutes to complete both steps.

Step 1. Agency Perspective

As an agency, discuss the following:

A. How many "lost souls" were produced (those who failed in treatment by the end of Round 2)?

B. With whom did you do the most referral work? Why?

C. How does your agency's success rate compare with its growth or decline as an agency?

D. Did your agency seem to offer quality care (that is, not straining the capacity of your service unit) or did your agency opt for growth through more clients?

Step 2. Participant Perspective

As a total group, discuss the following:

A. Were the assumptions upon which the simulation is based "real" in relation to the world of agency life?

B. What was the most confusing part of the simulation?

C. Which agency seemed the most successful? Why?

D. With which agencies did you prefer to work? Why?

E. To what extent did the state hospital serve as a "dumping ground" for certain types of patients?

F. How do the agency survival activities in the simulation relate to the concepts of organizational exchange?

REFERENCES

Levine, S., & White, P. E. Exchange as a conceptual framework for the study of interorganizational relationships. In Y. Hasenfeld & R. A. English (Eds.), Human service organizations. Ann Arbor, Mich.: University of Michigan Press, 1974.

RELATED READINGS

Benson, J. K., Kunce, J. T., Thompson, C. A., & Allen, D. L. Sociological study of an interorganizational network, Research Service no. 6. Columbia, Mo.: Regional Rehabilitation Research Institute, University of Missouri, Columbia, 1973.

Bloedorn, J. C., MacLatchie, E. B., Friedlander, W., & Wedemeyer, J. M. Designing social service systems. Chicago: American Public Welfare Association, 1970.

Mikulecky, T. J. (Ed.). Human services integration. Washington, D. C.: American Society for Public Administration, 1974.

Perlman, R. Consumers and social services. New York: John Wiley and Sons, 1975.

Rosenberg, M., & Brody, R. Systems serving people: A break-through in service delivery. Cleveland, Ohio: Case Western Reserve University, 1974.

7

HANPLAN: HANOVER COUNTY MENTAL HEALTH ASSOCIATION
CONDUCTS A COMMUNITY NEEDS ASSESSMENT

Beth Sodec

I. INTRODUCTION

Local mental health associations which involve lay and
professional people are an important part of the mental health service
system. Such associations can serve as a vital link between the
community and the agencies, providing a communitywide viewpoint and a
forum for the exchange of ideas. Local mental health associations are
chapters of the National Association for Mental Health and are funded
through membership fees, grants, and United Fund allocations. Many
local mental health associations across the country work on the
following priorities: (1) improved care and treatment of mental
hospital patients; (2) aftercare and rehabilitation services;
(3) special services for mentally ill children; and (4) comprehensive
community mental health services.

Many mental health associations are relatively small
organizations with an executive director and several support staff.
The board of directors of such voluntary organizations work through
such subcommittees as fund raising, program planning, community
education, etc. Most associations do not operate mental health
services except when new innovative programs are developed as
experiments. If such programs are successful, they are usually
transferred to existing agencies.

Mental health associations have traditionally contributed to increased public understanding of mental health problems through community education programs and legislative advocacy. The executive director of a mental health association should be skilled as a program planner, organizer, fundraiser, lobbyist, group worker, public relations specialist, and administrator.

II. GOAL AND ENABLING OBJECTIVES

Goal:

> To acquaint participants with the dynamics of executive-board relationships in a mental health association in relationship to determining community needs.

Enabling Objectives:

1. To teach participants the techniques of needs assessment.

2. To acquaint participants with goalsetting within an organization.

3. To teach participants to develop program priorities and service alternatives based on needs assessment.

4. To involve participants in resolving disagreements between the executive and the board of directors.

III. PROCEDURES

FRAME I - Assessing Community Needs

  Step 1. Reviewing Existing Data and Selecting an Approach
      (Read before beginning simulation)
  Step 2. Presenting Selections (40 minutes)
  Step 3. Analyzing Data (30 minutes)
  Step 4. Developing Human Needs Statements (20 minutes)
  Step 5. Debriefing (30 minutes)

FRAME II - Setting Goals

  Step 1. Assigning Roles (10 minutes)
  Step 2. Determining Goals (30 minutes)
  Step 3. Suggestion of Additional Goals (10 minutes)
  Step 4. Rank Ordering Goals (20 minutes)
  Step 5. Debriefing (20 minutes)

FRAME III - Developing Service Priorities

  Step 1. Developing Alternatives (15 minutes)
  Step 2. Choosing Among Alternatives (30 minutes)
  Step 3. The Board Meeting (30 minutes)
  Step 4. Debriefing (30 minutes)

FRAME I

ASSESSING COMMUNITY NEEDS

The Hanover County Mental Health Association has been experiencing hard times. During the last two years its membership and activities declined to the point that the association existed in name only. During the last six months, however, the new executive director, Claire Hanson, has worked hard and is reviving the association. She has applied for and received a $10,000 grant with which to conduct a needs assessment for Hanover County within the next nine months. The objectives of this study, according to the grant application, are:

1. To identify the major unmet mental health needs within Hanover County, and the expressed demand for care which is not being met by existing services;

2. Based on the findings from the needs assessment study, to develop service proposals to be presented to funding bodies such as the local United Fund, community mental health center, or state or federal agencies;

3. To provide hard data to be used by community agencies in developing their priorities for service;

4. To stimulate the involvement in needs assessment of interested lay and professional persons to promote community efforts in implementing the service proposals.

Conducting a needs assessment is a major undertaking. Accordingly, Ms. Hanson has recruited several graduate students from the local university to serve their internships with the association. These students will serve as staff for both planning and implementing the needs assessment study.

Step 1. Reviewing Existing Data and Selecting an Approach (Read before beginning simulation)

For this step, all participants should work alone in preparation for working in small planning groups of six in Step 2. Each participant should review Claire Hanson's memo on page 237 which defines and describes five approaches to needs assessment. Each participant should also review the description of current mental health services and the demographic data regarding Hanover County which is attached to Ms. Hanson's memo.

Based on the review, each participant should select the needs assessment approach or combination of approaches which seems best. In this case, "best" is defined as:

--appropriate to the goals of the study;

--does not exceed the time limit of nine months;

--does not exceed the monetary limit of $10,000.

After reviewing the following pages, write the approach, or combination of approaches, which <u>you</u> think is the best and indicate at least three reasons for your selection.

<u>Approach Selected</u>   <u>Justification (Reasons)</u>

#1 _____   _____

                                     _____

                                     _____

#2 _____   _____

                                     _____

                                     _____

#3 _____   _____

                                     _____

                                     _____

M E M O R A N D U M

TO: Planning Staff

FROM: Claire Hanson, Executive Director

RE: Community Needs Assessment

Attached is a summary of an article on the different approaches to needs assessment. Before undertaking a discussion of approaches, however, I feel it is important that we all share a common understanding of the purpose of a community needs assessment. For our situation, the needs assessment process, regardless of approach taken, is an attempt to enumerate the needs of the people living in our community by completing four steps:

1. identifying the extent and kinds of needs of people within a community; then

2. evaluating systematically the community's existing programs; then

3. comparing the community's needs to the existing service patterns of the community's programs to discover where the "gaps" are; and finally

4. planning new programs based on the needs assessment.

In our case, we are obviously talking about only those aspects of human need and community programs which relate to mental health.

Before setting out to collect data which will enable us to proceed through the above four steps, however, we must ask ourselves the following questions. The answers to these questions have a direct bearing on which approach to needs assessment we will choose.

1. What do we want/need to know about human needs and community programs? And why do we want to know this?

2. What useful data sources already exist at the local, state, and federal levels?

3. What data will we have to collect ourselves?

4. What will the data collection cost?

5. How long will it take to complete?

6. Which of the available needs assessment approaches will be most efficient for our purposes?

On the following pages are descriptions of the five basic approaches to needs assessment (Part I): the key informants approach; the community forum approach; the rates-under-treatment approach; the social indicators approach; and the field survey approach. I have included also a time and cost estimate for each approach.

Also attached is a description of the current mental health services (Part II) and demographic data regarding Hanover County which will be useful for the social indicators approach (Part III).

PART I. FIVE APPROACHES TO COMMUNITY NEEDS ASSESSMENT

This summary is adapted from G. J. Warheit, R. A. Bell, and J. J. Schwab, Planning for change: Needs assessment approaches, NIMH Grant 15900-05 S-1, 1974.

1. KEY INFORMANTS APPROACH

Key informants are persons who are knowledgeable, both in terms of statistical data and political structure, about the community's needs and service utilization patterns. Persons normally selected as key informants for our area would include public officials, the administrative and program personnel in the health and welfare organizations of the community, health purveyors from the public and private sectors (physicians and public health nurses), and personnel from vocational rehabilitation agencies, guidance clinics, and other health agencies.

After you decide what you want/need to know (or set the objectives of the assessment) and you select the key informants, the next step is to construct a questionnaire or interview schedule. This instrument is administered generally through a personal interview, since such a method permits face-to-face contact, a free exchange of ideas, and a high response rate.

Advantages: 1. Simple and inexpensive

                2. Permits input from varying perspectives

                3. Helps to open lines of communication among
                    human service agencies

                4. Helps to increase communication, which may
                    lead to greater community involvement

Disadvantages: 1. Built-in bias of informants based on individual
                    or organizational priorities

                2. Reflects personal opinions only; lacks hard
                    data

Estimated Cost: $3,000

Estimated Time: 2 months

2. COMMUNITY FORUM APPROACH

A community forum is a group of people which includes both key informants and persons from the general population. It is conducted by holding a series of public meetings to which all residents are invited, in which people express their beliefs about the needs and service patterns of the community.

Advantages:
1. Easy to arrange and inexpensive
2. Permits input from varying segments of the community
3. Identifies interested citizens for future involvement

Disadvantages:
1. Difficult to gain representative attendance at meetings
2. May become a grievance session dominated by one group
3. May contribute to rising expectations about new services
4. Results in impressionistic data which is difficult to analyze

Estimated Cost: $4,000

Estimated Time: 2 months

3. RATES-UNDER-TREATMENT APPROACH

This approach involves a description of persons who have used the services of the health and welfare agencies of a community. The underlying assumption is that community needs can be estimated from a sample of individuals who have received care or treatment. This approach has been widely used to estimate the health needs and service patterns of consumers.

Advantages:
1. Readily available and inexpensive data
2. Increases communication among service providers
3. Increases awareness of community needs

Disadvantages:
1. Problems in guaranteeing confidentiality of data
2. Problems in determining representative sample
3. Difficult to project number of unserved people

4. Fails to account for those served outside the community

5. Assumes that all those who need care are receiving it already--that there is no untapped population of potential clients

Estimated Cost: $5,000

Estimated Time: 5 months

4. SOCIAL INDICATORS APPROACH

Social indicators are inferences from descriptive statistics found in public records and reports. Needs are inferred from these social indicators, particularly those statistics which are highly correlated with persons in need. Such statistics would be housing patterns, age, race, sex, income; crime rates, substance abuse, family patterns, morbidity and mortality rates, housing conditions (particularly substandard housing and overcrowding), accessibility to services and economic conditions.

Advantages: 1. Data already exists and is inexpensive

2. Data can be compared with other communities

3. A wide range of data is valuable in compiling an index of need

Disadvantages: 1. Indicators are only indirect measures of need

2. Data may reflect class bias (e.g., divorce rates)

3. Data reflects limited sources (census data doesn't reflect social views)

Estimated Cost: $3,000

Estimated Time: 4 months

5. FIELD SURVEY APPROACH

A survey is a poll conducted with a representative sample of the population of the community. The most frequently used methods are interview schedules or questionnaires composed of items constructed to gain information from respondents regarding their health, social well-being, and the patterns of care or service being received. The instruments can be administered in person or through the mail.

Advantages: 1. Scientifically valid and reliable data
                     2. Yields specific information about individual
                         needs and service utilization
                     3. If households are units of analysis, data
                         from other family members is available
Disadvantages: 1. Survey methods are expensive (interview or
                         postal costs)
                     2. Respondents are often reluctant to share
                         sensitive information
                     3. Nonreturn rates of questionnaire may make
                         results suspect
Estimated Cost: $7,000
Estimated Time: 8 months

PART II. HANOVER COUNTY MENTAL HEALTH SERVICES

Inpatient

Mental health resources for families and children are limited in
Hanover County. Hanover General Hospital provides emergency
psychiatric care to nonspecialized populations. Hanover General has no
mental health geriatric program, yet it has many patients over 65.
Hanover General does not have a day-treatment program, nor is there
such a facility in the county. Some aftercare services are available
for discharged psychiatric patients in an outpatient clinic through the
hospital and through the Hanover Community Mental Health Center, but
there is little evidence of aftercare planning in either facility.
Most of the 24 psychiatric beds at Hanover General are for private
paying patients with use of social service, clinical psychology, or
occupational therapy and no substantial evidence of a "therapeutic
community."

Outpatient Psychiatric Clinic

Hanover County's Community Mental Health Center provides the
outpatient services in the community. The clinic is, at present,
heavily burdened and understaffed, especially in certain program areas.
There is currently no crisis intervention service although suicide and
attempted suicide pose major problems. Outpatient services for

children and adolescents are severely limited, as are alcoholism, drug, and geriatric services.

Alcoholism Services

1. Private treatment - Available data reveal that a small proportion of the alcoholic population receive psychotherapeutic or counseling assistance from private practitioners.
2. Hanover General Hospital tends not to admit alcoholics or admits them with reluctance and frequently under other diagnoses.
3. State mental hospitals provide relatively short-term care (averaging less than two months). This resource is usually used in the absence of less appropriate facilities.
4. Alcoholics Anonymous - Generally considered inadequate but active in the community.
5. Salvation Army - Men's Social Service provides adequate diet and shelter plus occupational and social rehabilitation through collection, renovation, and sale of discarded materials provided by the community.
6. Hanover County Community Mental Health Center provides counseling although facilities are severely limited. The county has no detoxification facility other than Hanover General.

Drug Abuse Services

1. Hanover County Community Mental Health Center provides limited services.
2. Hanover General Hospital provides emergency services, somewhat reluctantly. Staff is untrained in handling drug crises.

The Schools

Three-fourths of all children in the county are enrolled in public and private school systems which lack programs for the emotionally handicapped. The two schools which have programs for the emotionally handicapped are both elementary and these are very limited. Particular note should be made of the scarcity of mental health personnel in the schools (e.g., school social workers, psychologists, counselors, and so forth). Very little coordination exists between the schools and the community mental health services.

Other Community Resources

Community resources are limited. There is a serious shortage of facilities for diagnostic and treatment services for children. There are currently no residential or day-treatment centers for children and adolescents.

PART III. HANOVER COUNTY DEMOGRAPHIC DATA

Hanover County includes a population of 205,000 including the city of Hanover and its suburban districts. Over the past 15 years, Hanover has slowly changed from a small town to a more cosmopolitan city, a change which has not been viewed favorably by all of its residents. Hanover has no large or heavy industries. It is generally a commercial center with offices for the factories established in surrounding areas located within the city. A number of small light manufacturers are located throughout the city and a number of maintenance and public service firms are concentrated within the city. This economic and occupational structure has contributed to an almost equal number of blue-collar workers and clerical, managerial, and professional workers.

A recent survey completed by the State Division of Mental Health should provide a clearer understanding of the community and its problems. Data from this survey are listed below and on the following page.

1. Socioeconomic Characteristics

Percentage unemployed	8.2	Percentage of population living in crowded housing	12.1
Median education level	11.4	Percentage of population - black	19.7
Percentages of families below the poverty level	18.8	Percentage of population - dependent aged	17.1
Median income level	$5219	Percentage of population - dependent youth	67.0

2. Mental Health Resources

Total Expenditure, State and Local	$2,169,340.00
Expenditure per Person, State and Local	$ 9.95

3. Selected Social Problem Indicators of Hanover County

Criteria	Rate Per 100,000	Rank*
Admissions to Child Welfare Services	157.6	15
Admissions to State Mental Hospitals	76.3	11
Admissions to Alcoholic Rehabilitation Center	22.5	4
Admissions to Youth Correctional Schools	53.2	2
Prisoners Received--Division of Corrections	36.4	20
Suicides for 2-Year Period	10.6	18
Residents in Retardation Training School	55.9	21
Admissions to Nursing Home	60.2	8
Admissions to Drug Abuse Rehabilitation	15.0	13

*Rank--indicates the numerical ranking of this social indicator among 42 counties in this state.

<u>Step 2. Presenting Selections</u> (40 minutes)

In the first part of this step, each small group of six participants will have 30 minutes to discuss the options identified by each participant and then reach consensus in order to present its choice for needs assessment and its justification to the other groups. Before making the presentation, review the following criteria:

1. Will the survey approach(es) fall within the grant budget of $10,000?

2. Will the survey approach(es) be completed within the nine-month grant period?

3. Will the survey approach(es) yield valid and reliable data as to the mental health needs of our community?

4. Will the survey approach(es) yield data which will fulfill the stated purposes of the study?

5. How will the approach(es) serve additional purposes, such as helping to educate the community about mental health needs?

When you all have chosen the approach(es) which the planning staff of the Hanover County Mental Health Association will take in conducting a needs assessment, write that choice below.

Approach(es)	Time Needed	Total Cost
_____	_____	_____
_____	_____	_____
_____	_____	_____

Identify one member of your group to make a <u>brief</u> presentation on the approach(es) selected and the justification for each. Your instructor will give your group a number and then list your selections on a blackboard.

Step 3. Analyzing Data (30 minutes)

While it would take considerable time under normal circumstances to collect the data, for this simulation the data has already been collected. It is now time for the planning staff to analyze that data to develop initial statements of need.

Your instructor will give each small planning group only the data which was collected by the needs assessment approach(es) that were chosen by your group. Each small group is to work by itself to develop three major findings of needs which exist in Hanover County by completing the following forms.

UNMET NEED #1

1. Unmet need, according to data gathered during needs assessment:

_____

_____

2. Refer to data originally provided for you in Ms. Hanson's memo on needs assessment. Does this shed any light on this need? Is the need modified by the original data? If so, restate the need.

_____

_____

3. Which agency in Hanover County might be meeting this need and to what extent? (Refer again to Ms. Hanson's original memo.) Agency meeting need and percentage of need being met (if none, write "none"):

_____

_____

4. Final statement of unmet need:

_____

_____

Justification for this statement: _____

_____

_____

UNMET NEED #2

1. Unmet need, according to data gathered during needs assessment:

   _____

   _____

2. Refer to data originally provided for you in Ms. Hanson's memo on
   needs assessment. Does this shed any light on this need? Is the
   need modified by the original data? If so, restate the need.

   _____

   _____

3. Which agency in Hanover County might be meeting this need and to
   what extent? (Refer again to Ms. Hanson's original memo.)
   Agency meeting need and percentage of need being met (if none,
   write "none"):

   _____

   _____

4. Final statement of unmet need:

   _____

   _____

   Justification for this statement: _____

   _____

   _____

UNMET NEED #3

1. Unmet need, according to data gathered during needs assessment:

    _____

    _____

2. Refer to data originally provided for you in Ms. Hanson's memo on needs assessment. Does this shed any light on this need? Is the need modified by the original data? If so, restate the need.

    _____

    _____

3. Which agency in Hanover County might be meeting this need and to what extent? (Refer again to Ms. Hanson's original memo.) Agency meeting need and percentage of need being met (if none, write "none"):

    _____

    _____

4. Final statement of unmet need:

    _____

    _____

    Justification for this statement: _____

    _____

    _____

Step 4. Developing Human Needs Statements (20 minutes)

In this step, each small planning group should make a very brief verbal presentation of its three major needs statements to the other groups. As the statements are being presented, each participant should write the statements on a separate sheet of paper. After all groups have made their presentation, work together in your small group to combine any statements that are similar and transfer your final list onto the Preliminary List of Human Needs Statements.

When you have a final list of statements (in which none of the statements duplicates another statement), rank order each statement. Use "1" for the most important, "2" for the next most important, etc. The executive director will later present this list and your ranking to the board of directors.

PRELIMINARY LIST OF HUMAN NEEDS STATEMENTS

Ranking

_____   Statement A. _____

           _____

_____   Statement B. _____

           _____

_____   Statement C. _____

           _____

_____   Statement D. _____

           _____

_____   Statement E. _____

           _____

_____   Statement F. _____

           _____

_____   Statement G. _____

           _____

_____   Statement H. _____

           _____

_____   Statement I. _____

           _____

Step 5. Debriefing (30 minutes)

Working within your small planning groups, answer the following questions:

1. How realistic is the final list of unmet needs?

2. Was there any system used to develop the ranking? Was any justification cited?

3. Do you feel that the data which was gathered in the needs assessment survey is realistic? That is, in the real world, would the same type of data be gathered (in terms of specificity, completeness, etc.)?

4. In hindsight would you have chosen a different needs assessment approach? If so, which one?

If your instructor chooses to debrief the experiences of all participants in one large group, it is helpful to address the following questions to which all participants can relate:

1. How did your group reach consensus and what factors contributed to your group process?

2. How comprehensive is each needs assessment approach and what problems does each approach create?

3. How adequate was the data used by your group and how could the quality of the data be improved?

4. What are the problems inherent in translating the data into needs statements?

5. How should the mental health needs of a community be defined?

FRAME II

SETTING GOALS

Claire Hanson has recommended the scheduling of a special meeting of the board of directors in order to reexamine and consider both the purposes and goals of the association. With dissension increasing over the past few months around the directions that the association should take, this meeting has been called in order to clarify directions and hopefully gain commitment to the results of the needs assessment study. Ms. Hanson hopes that this meeting can serve to unify the board in purpose and commitment. Prior to today's meeting, Ms. Hanson had asked the education committee to prepare a list of association goals to be the framework for discussion at the board meeting. The questions seem to be: What should our goals be? What is our association's role in the community?

Step 1. Assigning Roles (10 minutes)

Your instructor will divide you into groups of six and assign roles within each small group. The roles are:
- --Claire Hanson, the executive director of the HCMHA;
- --Gerald Davis, the chairman of the board and a business executive;
- --John Starnes, a physician;
- --Carolyn Reardon, a retired school counselor;
- --Betty Owen, an attorney;
- --Michael Daily, a banker.

Every participant should read the following two pages, which describe the duties of both the board of directors and the executive director. Then, read your role description on the following pages. Read only your role description.

Responsibilities of the Board of Directors

The duties and responsibilities of the board of directors can be summarized as follows:

1. Establishes and maintains the legal or corporate existence of the association.

2. Oversees the management of all property and affairs of the association.

3. Identifies the mental health needs of the citizens.

4. Decides on desired action, depending on resources. Determines necessary priorities, policies, and organizational procedures with regard to the organization and its relationship to other components.

5. Acquires and allocates the volunteer and staff manpower to carry out the desired program. Establishes conditions of employment of staff members. Is responsible for the selection of the executive director.

6. Acquires and allocates the financial resources to carry out the desired program and the shared support of the division and/or the national level program. Is accountable for the expenditure of funds.

7. Conducts periodic evaluation of the association's program and operations.

8. Interprets the work of the mental health association to the public.

9. Inspires confidence in the program because of the competence of the board members as active trustees of the association.

10. Provides continuity of experienced leadership so that officer and staff changes will not weaken the effectiveness of the association.

Responsibilities of the Executive Director

The executive director is employed by the board of directors. Additional staff may be employed by the executive director. The duties and responsibilities of the executive director can be summarized as follows:

1. Oversees the implementation of the objectives, policies, and programs established by the board of directors.

2. Facilitates the functioning of the board of directors by keeping the board well informed on community and mental health needs, association activities, and progress in the carrying out of the association's programs and policies.

3. Recommends for board consideration needed policies, impending program and financial needs, and alternatives for meeting those needs.

4. Renders professional and technical assistance to the board and committees to facilitate their functioning.

5. Procures technical expertise as required.

6. Represents, when appropriate, the association.

7. Relates the association's activities to other groups and governmental bodies.

8. Administers the association's office and office activities, including: standard office services to the elected officers, board, and committees; assistance to the general public and other agencies; management of the association's financial affairs as designated.

Role-Play Instructions for <u>Claire Hanson</u>, Executive Director

During the past several months you have clearly antagonized several members of the board whose view of the role of the mental health association is less change-oriented than yours. It is clear to you that during tonight's meeting you must work <u>toward reconciling splintered factions among the board while at the same time helping the board members realize the need to make the association a viable force in the community</u>. You have a strong awareness of services currently available, and the pressing extent of unmet needs. You are anxious to incorporate the statements from the needs assessment into the association's goal statements. In tonight's meeting you will play a facilitative role in helping board members adopt a statement of goals.

Role-Play Instructions for <u>Gerald Davis</u>, Board Chairman

Although you are identified as a conservative member of the board, you are really too preoccupied with numerous business and civic interests to be a strong leader in the association. The Hanover County Mental Health Association has, in fact, been only a peripheral interest of yours. You are quite concerned about not alienating community agencies by pushing too intently. Also, you are somewhat embarrassed about representing the mental health association as you still harbor some unclear notions about mental health in general. You have been unhappy about Ms. Hanson's strong push to create a forceful organization, but your interest in the association has really been only superficial; thus you have not strongly opposed her. You generally strive to <u>keep board meetings orderly, play down controversial issues, and "soft pedal" the association</u> to other community groups.

Goal Preference: Information and Education

Role-Play Instructions for <u>John Starnes</u>, Board Member

      You have been a member of the Hanover County Mental Health Association since its inception in 1952. You have been satisfied with the association over the past years and have felt that it has served its purpose through recruiting volunteers to work at the nearby state mental hospital and through sponsoring occasional public information forums on mental health issues. You are quite angry about Ms. Hanson's efforts to press the association forward, preferring to maintain a low-key profile. You think that the needs assessment was a huge waste of money. You are also skeptical about the recent trends toward community care, such as halfway houses, believing that care of the mentally ill is best left in the physician's (psychiatrist's) hands. You believe that the field of mental health has been invaded by radicals with "street theories." <u>You see the role of the association as strictly educational and informational</u>. You may choose to become more angry or mollified, depending on how Claire Hanson responds to your concerns.

      Goal Preferences: Information and Education

                             Increased volunteer services for state hospital residents

Role-Play Instructions for <u>Carolyn Reardon</u>, Board Member

You have been a board member of the Hanover County Mental Health Association for just one year and believe that the association could be much more viable than it has been in the past. As a member of the community for many years and as a retired school counselor, you are especially aware of the community's problems, particularly as they relate to school children and adolescents. <u>One of your main objectives as an association member is to work for improvements in mental health services for children and youth.</u> You have noted problems increasing dramatically over the past several years without an increase in available resources. It is your belief that the community is not aware of the extent of unmet needs and the lack of resources. In general you feel that Ms. Hanson's leadership has been effective, although you are concerned about recent dissension among the board.

Goal Preferences: To promote special services for children and youth

To promote alcoholism services which represents a new goal

Role-Play Instructions for <u>Betty Owen</u>, Board Member

You are a well-respected member of the community, an attorney, and
a strong advocate of improved mental health services. You have been a
strong and stable member of the Hanover County Mental Health
Association for a number of years and, like Claire Hanson, you are
eager to see the association become a <u>significant force in the
community</u>, especially in view of the great need for services within the
community. You are aware that certain board members are not eager for
and perhaps are threatened by change and thus seek a firm but
facilitative manner in presenting your views and helping others clarify
theirs. You are especially interested in promoting alcoholism
services, increased services for the elderly, and lobbying efforts with
the legislature.

> Goal Preferences: To promote alcoholism services
>
> To promote services for the elderly
> (submit as new goal)
>
> To promote lobbying efforts

Role-Play Instructions for <u>Michael Daily</u>, Board Member

Like John Starnes, you prefer a low-key profile for the Hanover
County Mental Health Association. You do have one very strong program
interest: job counseling, training or retraining, and sheltered
workshops for recovering mental patients. You are firmly convinced
that work is the best therapy for most people, and <u>helping the mentally
ill become functioning individuals certainly reduces the tax drain.</u>
Your unexpressed belief is that the mentally ill have simply chosen a
method of avoiding work and responsibility. You are in favor of
individuals "pulling themselves up by their bootstraps" and
"straightening themselves up." No nonsense. You also favor halfway
houses and foster homes with a strong vocational program thrust.

> Goal Preference: To promote job training and vocationally
> oriented halfway houses

Step 2. Determining Goals (30 minutes)

The board chairman, Gerald Davis, should call the meeting to order. Each board member will find a random listing of the goals of the Hanover County Mental Health Association below. The purpose of tonight's meeting is to decide on a list of goals to guide the association. To get the meeting started, Chairman Davis requests that each member, in turn, share with the board his/her view of which goal or goals should be of major concern to the association and what his/her views are regarding the most important purposes of the association. After each board member has presented his/her views, Chairman Davis should lead a general discussion focused on clarifying the perspectives of everyone present. Then Davis temporarily suspends discussion so that each board member can rank (1 = most important) the following goals which were carried over from last year.

THE GOALS AND PURPOSES OF THE HCMHA

Individual Ranking		Group Ranking
_____	To provide increased volunteer services for residents in the state hospital	_____
_____	To work through the state legislature to lobby for improved care and treatment for patients at the state hospital	_____
_____	To educate and inform the public and special groups about problems, needs, and association activities	_____
_____	To provide reliable information on available mental health services and facilities within our community	_____
_____	To work for the development within our community of a halfway house and more foster homes for recovering mental patients	_____
_____	To work with state hospital staff in developing improved care and treatment for the mentally ill	_____
_____	To work with community groups in developing special services for troubled young children and their families	_____
_____	To work for the development of adequate job counseling, training or retraining, and sheltered workshops for recovering mental patients	_____

Addition #1 _____   _____

_____

Addition #2 _____   _____

_____

Addition #3 _____   _____

_____

Step 3. Suggestion of Additional Goals (10 minutes)

After a general discussion of the currently slated goals, Davis requests that each board member suggest additional goals derived from the recently completed needs assessment (review Step 4 in Frame I) in terms of each member's orientation to current problems of the community and the association. Consensus should be reached on no more than three additional goals to be placed in the space at the bottom of the previous page. While Claire Hanson develops her own rankings, she does not share them with the group.

Step 4. Rank Ordering Goals (20 minutes)

As a final effort in tonight's meeting, Davis suggests that consensus be reached on a rank ordering of a composite slate of goals which will guide the future decisions and activities for the Hanover County Mental Health Association. The composite set of goals should include the goals already listed as well as additional goals agreed upon by the board. Adoption of a set of goals agreeable to the board requires a majority vote of all board members. Space for recording the final revised list of goals is found to the right of the list in Step 2.

<u>Step 5. Debriefing</u> (20 minutes)

Staying with the group within which you role-played, answer the following questions:

1. How big a role did the needs assessment information play in the setting and ranking of goals?

2. How realistic were the roles? Do you feel that most members of an executive board of a mental health association would act and feel as these members did?

3. If you had been Claire Hanson, how would you have conducted yourself in that meeting?

4. How critical are goal statements to the actual operation of an organization?

FRAME III

DEVELOPING SERVICE PRIORITIES

The meeting of the executive board is over and the goals for the Hanover County Mental Health Association have been set for the next year. Ms. Hanson has returned to her planning staff (the group of graduate students) and has told them about the outcome of the meeting.

She and her planning staff must now work on developing suggested programs, based on the needs assessment survey's results.

Step 1. Developing Alternatives (15 minutes)

Now that the data have been analyzed and a list of human needs statements has been written and rank ordered, it is time for the staff to work on suggesting alternatives which could meet those needs.

Copy the five human needs statements which received the highest rankings (that is, 1 through 5) from Frame II. For each needs statement, brainstorm by thinking of all the possible service alternatives that could fulfill that need. Write them all down on the following page. The service alternatives need not be confined to those that could be implemented by the mental health association itself. (For example, one service alternative could be that the MHA would work with Agency X to create Service Y.)

ALTERNATIVE SERVICE PRIORITIES

Needs Statement   Service Alternatives

1. _____   _____

   _____   _____

   _____   _____

                                               _____

2. _____   _____

   _____   _____

   _____   _____

                                               _____

3. _____   _____

   _____   _____

   _____   _____

                                               _____

4. _____   _____

   _____   _____

   _____   _____

                                               _____

5. _____   _____

   _____   _____

   _____   _____

                                               _____

<u>Step 2. Choosing Among Alternatives</u> (30 minutes)

Now that you have brainstormed, it is time to begin to select which service alternative could best meet the unmet needs. For each needs statement, choose the one alternative that you as a group think is best. Some of the criteria by which you should be guided in your choices are:

--The program should probably be centered in the mental health association, as the MHA would have better control over it.

--Funding for the program should be available. (Suggest the estimated amount needed for the program and where it might be available.)

--Expertise for the program should be available.

On the following page, write down which alternative you have selected for each needs statement, who should do it, the percentage of the need that will be alleviated if it is done, how much you think it will cost, and where the money can be obtained.

Ms. Hanson will be presenting this to the board at their next meeting.

SERVICE PRIORITIES

Suggested Program	Percentage of Need	Who Should Do It	Estimated Cost	Possible Source of Funding
1.				
2.				
3.				
4.				
5.				

Step 3. The Board Meeting (30 minutes)

Your instructor will divide you into groups of six and within these groups assign you to one of the following roles:

--Claire Hanson, executive director;

--Gerald Davis, board chairman;

--John Starnes, board member and physician;

--Carolyn Reardon, board member and retired school counselor;

--Betty Owen, board member and attorney;

--Michael Daily, board member and banker.

Once each of you has read his/her role descriptions (do not read anyone else's), Gerald Davis will open the meeting. Each person will then state generally in which direction he/she would like to see the association move during the next two years. After this round-table discussion is completed, Mr. Davis will then open the floor for specific suggestions.

When your group has completed this step, wait for your instructor before proceeding to the next step.

Role Description for <u>Claire Hanson</u>, Executive Director

This meeting tonight will set the course of the mental health association for the next two years, and you are extremely anxious about its outcome. You very much want to see the needs assessment results implemented and you also very much want to keep your job. You know that several of the executive board members are irritated with you, as they feel you push too much for change.

Yet you can't help feeling that the data is so conclusive and the logic is so tight that the needs assessment just can't fail. You don't see how anyone could refute its findings. Accordingly, you will push with minimal input into the discussion for <u>adoption of the needs assessment results</u> as the direction the association should take for the next two years.

Role Description for <u>Gerald Davis</u>, Board Chairman

You received the package on needs assessment that Ms. Hanson sent you, but you just glanced over it. The mental health association has never been one of your top priorities. The only reason you're staying on the board is that it's less embarrassing for you to continue than it would be for you to resign.

You were mildly interested in the association's goals which it set before, and you think that they probably ought to be followed in the future. Yet your main concern is to <u>keep the meeting orderly and play down any controversial issues</u> that may arise. You want to develop a list of what the association will do over the next two years as quickly as possible and not drag the meeting out forever. (Remember to watch the clock since the meeting should last only 20 minutes.)

Role Description for <u>John Starnes</u>, Board Member

   As a physician and board member of the mental health association for the last 24 years, your ideas about what the association should and should not do are quite set. You feel that the association should be educational and informational, devoting itself to activities like recruiting volunteers to work at the nearby state mental hospital. The meeting in which the association set its goals was somewhat disturbing to you--you thought new and radical ideas were creeping in.

   You have thoroughly read the needs assessment package that Ms. Hanson sent you and you think it wasn't worth the paper it was printed on. The whole idea of needs assessment has enraged you--it is up to professionals, like physicians, to determine what the needs are and who shall meet them. The very fact of even thinking about a needs assessment implies that professionals are not doing their job, and you very much resent this slap in the face. Accordingly, you are intent upon making certain that the association <u>maintains its informational and educational functions to the exclusion of all other functions</u>, and you are quite prepared to be as vocal as necessary to make certain this comes to pass.

Role Description for <u>Carolyn Reardon</u>, Board Member

You are a retired school counselor and so are very interested in the problems of children and adolescents. You are fairly aware of the community's problems, so nothing in the needs assessment took you by surprise. You would have preferred that youth come out with a higher priority. You are willing to follow the recommendations that have been set forth by Ms. Hanson and her staff.

Ms. Hanson has not enjoyed all the support you feel she should have from the board. In order for her to get this support, however, you know that the dissension which exists on the board must be toned down. You perceive that there are many "but we've always done it this way" type of persons on the board. You think that you might be able to serve as a bridge between the new ideas espoused by Ms. Hanson and the older, conservative ideologies of most of the board members. If push comes to shove, however, you will support Ms. Hanson. Accordingly, your objectives for this meeting are <u>to implement the recommendations of the needs assessment study and perhaps even to bind together the warring factions on the board</u>.

Role Description for <u>Betty Owen</u>, Board Member

Having been an attorney in Hanover County for 30 years, you are well acquainted with the members of the board. Although you match several of them in age, you match very few of them in ideas. You feel that the association must become a more active force in the community, and you support Ms. Hanson and her ideas. You are not very sure of the needs assessment study, as you feel that its methodology is faulty: nowhere could you find what priority system was used in ranking the human needs statements. You'd like to have this question on methodology answered by Ms. Hanson.

You see the needs assessment as being a means to an end, the end being the association's becoming a significant force in the community. You think that the association could become such a force by promoting alcoholism services and/or increased services for the elderly. These two items are high on your personal list of priorities. Accordingly, you would like <u>to have your question on methodology answered and then develop the quickest and most forceful way the association can become a significant force in Hanover County</u>. You know that Dr. Starnes will disagree with you in your aims for the association. It is a battle you and he have fought many times; you do not hesitate to fight it again with him.

Role Description for <u>Michael Daily</u>, Board Member

You have read the needs assessment package and you do not agree at all with its service priorities. Your bases of disagreement are two. First, you agree with Dr. Starnes that the association should assume a low profile. Second, you believe that the cure for almost any ill is work. Work helps people become functional again and thus reduces the tax drain. Work also gets people out of the habit of looking to somebody else for help, instead of pulling themselves up by their bootstraps. It also weeds out the lazy imbeciles who shouldn't be supported by the government.

Although you don't agree with the service priorities, you do feel that Ms. Hanson has done a fairly adequate job on the needs assessment. This is the first businesslike thing she has done, and you'd like to congratulate her on producing some hard data rather than just giving you impressions and recitations from textbooks. You'd like to see the association keep its low profile during the next two years, primarily through <u>encouraging the establishment of job training and vocationally-oriented halfway houses</u>.

Step 4. Debriefing (30 minutes)

Answer the following questions in your whole group:

1. What were the results of each board meeting?

2. What was the match or fit between the recommended service priorities and the existing services in Hanover County noted in Frame I?

3. Did you feel that the needs assessment package was a "sure winner?" Did the people who criticized the needs assessment have any valid criticisms?

4. How did Claire Hanson try to influence others regarding her point of view? What would you have done, if you had been in her position?

5. What are some potential sources of strain between the executive director of a voluntary association and its lay board members? How can these best be handled?

RELATED READINGS

Bauer, R. A. (Ed.). <u>Social indicators</u>. Cambridge, Mass.: M. I. T. Press, 1966.

Blum, H. L. <u>Planning for health</u>. New York: Behavioral Publications, 1976.

Bradshaw, J. The concept of social need. In N. Gilbert and H. Specht (Eds.), <u>Planning for social welfare</u>. Englewood Cliffs, N. J.: Prentice-Hall, 1977.

Center for Social Research and Development, University of Denver. <u>Analysis and synthesis of needs assessment research in the field of human services</u>. Denver, Colo.: University of Denver, 1976.

Cox, F., Erlich, J., Rottman, J., & Tropman, J. E. <u>Tactics and techniques of community practice</u>. Itasca, Ill.: F. E. Peacock, 1977.

Epstein, I., & Tripodi, T. <u>Research techniques for program planning, monitoring, and evaluation</u>. New York: Columbia University Press, 1977.

Gilbert, N., & Specht, H. (Eds.). <u>Planning for social welfare</u>. Englewood Cliffs, N. J.: Prentice-Hall, 1977.

Institute for Social Service Planning, School of Social Work, University of North Carolina. <u>Problem analysis/need assessment: An expanding role for the local human service administrator</u>. Chapel Hill, N. C.: University of North Carolina, 1977.

Katz, D., Gutek, B. A., Kahn, R. L., & Barton, E. <u>Bureaucratic encounters: A pilot study in the evaluation of governmental services</u>. Ann Arbor, Mich.: University of Michigan Press, 1975.

National Institute of Mental Health. <u>Resource materials for community mental health program evaluation</u>, 2nd Ed. Washington, D. C.: U. S. Government Printing Office, 1977.

National Institute of Mental Health. <u>A working manual of simple program evaluation techniques for community mental health centers</u>. Washington, D. C.: U. S. Government Printing Office, 1971.

Thayer, R. Measuring need in the social services. In N. Gilbert and H. Specht (Eds.), <u>Planning for social welfare</u>. Englewood Cliffs, N. J.: Prentice-Hall, 1977.

The Research Group, Inc. <u>Techniques for needs assessment in social services planning</u>. Atlanta, Ga.: The Research Group, Inc., 1976.

The Research Group, Inc. <u>Report on the assessment of needs for social services in the state of Alabama</u>. Atlanta, Ga.: The Research Group, Inc., 1977.

Warheit, G. J., Bell, R. A., & Schwab, J. J. Planning for change: Needs assessment approach. Washington, D. C.: National Institute of Mental Health, 1978.

Webb, K., & Hatry, H. P. Obtaining citizens' feedback: The application of citizen surveys to local governments. Washington, D. C.: The Urban Institute, 1973.

8

HALFWAY: THE ADMINISTRATION OF

A PSYCHIATRIC HALFWAY HOUSE

Patricia Yancey Martin

I. INTRODUCTION

"Halfway" is a social simulation which places each participant in
the position of the executive director or a key staff person in a
psychiatric halfway house. It focuses on the need to integrate client
and community objectives in order to provide effective client services
while maintaining good community relations.

The setting is an average-size residential facility with promising
potential. It is, however, currently experiencing serious difficulties
regarding its relationship(s) with the community and the effectiveness
of its "client services." Attempting to resolve these problems through
group decision making is, we believe, both realistic and beneficial.
At a minimum it allows each team member to become actively involved in
a problem-solving endeavor and, in the process, to utilize his/her
experiences and abilities to the fullest.

"Halfway" is a simulation of a "typical" psychiatric halfway house
and is based on research data and case materials. As such, it is
obviously less than a perfect model of reality. However, it attempts
to represent certain aspects of real halfway houses, particularly as
related to decision-making processes around the issues of:

1. Program planning;

2. Staffing;

3. Financing;
4. Client placement and follow up;
5. Client admissions;
6. Community relations.

A key feature of "Halfway" is that participants must discover for themselves the range of problems related to halfway house management. As in real life, some of the forces to be dealt with in the simulation are such that participants have almost complete control over them, such as the roles and responsibilities of staff members and the type of treatment program which clients will be offered. Other factors, however, are only partially under the control of staff members, such as the successful job placement of residents and the climate of neighborhood opinion.

II. GOAL AND ENABLING OBJECTIVES

Goal:

> To acquaint participants with the issues and skills necessary to administer a halfway house.

Enabling Objectives:

1. Demonstrate ability to identify important issues and/or problems in the administration of a halfway house.

2. Develop skills in identifying program goals and establishing program priorities.

3. Develop skills in program planning to implement goals.

4. Develop skills in dealing with conflicting, contradictory, and/or hostile demands from the environment of a halfway house program.

5. Gain knowledge of the procedures by which an administrator of a halfway house induces and supports staff to participate in collective goal setting, program planning, and decision making.

6. Gain knowledge of the inherent conflict between effective service provision to clients and financial solvency of an agency.

7. Gain knowledge of the role and function of the executive committee and chairman of the board of the board of directors of a halfway house program.

III. <u>PROCEDURES</u>

BACKGROUND FRAME - Bridge Place: The Case Situation (Read before beginning simulation)

FRAME I - Relationship of Bridge Place to Other Agencies

- Step 1. Setting the Scene (5 minutes)
- Step 2. What Is the Problem? (15 minutes)
- Step 3. Developing a Solution (30 minutes)
- Step 4. Debriefing (25 minutes)

FRAME II - Prioritizing Issues and Task Force Planning

- Step 1. Getting Ready (5 minutes)
- Step 2. Wrestling with the Issues (20 minutes)
- Step 3. Task Force Planning for Implementation (30 minutes)

FRAME III - Decision Making in the Context of Daily Pressures

- Step 1. Presenting Suggestions (15 minutes)
- Step 2. Dealing with Daily Pressures (30 minutes)
- Step 3. Debriefing (30 minutes)

FRAME IV - Relationship of Bridge Place to the Public

- Step 1. Reaction of the Executive Director (20 minutes)
- Step 2. Reaction of the Board (30 minutes)
- Step 3. Debriefing (10 minutes)

FRAME V - Changing the Program

- Step 1. Devising Plans (20 minutes)
- Step 2. Sharing Plans (10 minutes)
- Step 3. Debriefing (45 minutes)

BACKGROUND FRAME

BRIDGE PLACE: THE CASE SITUATION

Bridge Place has now been in operation for two full years. It is
the only psychiatric halfway house in the city of Campbell and
currently houses 22 residents of both sexes. Residents are allowed
to stay at Bridge Place for a maximum of one year, during which time
they are expected to obtain employment and to become relatively
independent. Each resident is encouraged to handle his or her personal
affairs and to participate in recreational, educational, and cultural
activities in the community.

About three years ago, a number of interested citizens in
Campbell (and in surrounding Dibbs County) established Bridge Place as
a "halfway house" for ex-hospital and prehospital psychiatric patients.
These citizens, many of whom were members of the local mental health
association, intended that Bridge Place would be an independent,
nonprofit local agency. To help get Bridge Place off the ground, a
number of these persons assumed positions as members of the board of
directors. The board currently has 12 members, including two
physicians, one psychologist, a social worker, the president of the
Dibbs County Mental Health Association, a minister, a teacher, two
businessmen, a former mental hospital patient (now a sales clerk), the
local county sheriff, and the society editor of the local newspaper.
The first official act by the board of directors was to hire an
executive director for Bridge Place. They chose David Thomas because
of his mental health experience, pleasing personality, and his record
of being a hard worker and good fundraiser.

Starting with a small staff consisting of himself, a
secretary-bookkeeper (one-half time), a social worker, and a
rehabilitation counselor, David steadily expanded the program. From a
modest beginning of 10 residents and $3\frac{1}{2}$ full-time staff during the
first year, David saw the house grow to handle over 20 residents with
$6\frac{1}{2}$ full-time staff, plus a regularly consulting psychiatrist and a
physician on call. Further, the budget has grown from expenditures in
the first year of $45,000 to expenditures in the upcoming year of
$69,300 (see Figure 1). David proved a shrewd fundraiser and was

successful in getting financial aid from the United Fund, Dibbs County Mental Health Association, Mill Valley Mental Health Clinic, and a research and demonstration grant from the State Department of Mental Health. Expenses, however, are expected to exceed known revenues in the upcoming year. This problem could become a major issue for a new executive director.

The rapid increase in the number of residents at Bridge Place was made possible both by the size of the house, purchased with the aid of the two businessmen on the board of directors, and by the increase in number of staff. Bridge Place is a comfortable, Victorian mansion in an older section of the city of Campbell. It has three stories. Men are housed on the third floor and women on the second, while the first floor serves as the dining-living-recreational-laundry sector for general resident use. Ed Simms, the current resident manager, has a bedroom on the first floor, and the executive director has a small office suite (including a conference room which "doubles" as the residents' card/game room) nearby.

The physical location of Bridge Place is excellent for public transportation services; thus residents are able to get to their jobs, go shopping, etc., without problems. Further, although the neighborhood is old--and beginning to deteriorate--many families are still in the area and the neighborhood is considered to be quite safe.

The Residents

The criteria for the intake of residents are: referral by a hospital, clinic, agency, or psychiatrist because of emotional or mental disability; between the ages of 21 and 45; able to meet basic financial obligations; and moving toward employment. Although psychiatric halfway houses have traditionally served posthospital residents only, Bridge Place reflects the current trend toward increasing acceptance of prehospital residents.

Of the 22 current residents, 10 were previously hospitalized for a year or less, 7 for one to three years, and 4 for four or more years. One resident has never been hospitalized but, unless he is able to "improve" while at Bridge Place, he will soon be hospitalized. Upon release from the state mental hospital (in nearby Vegas County),

Figure 1

ANTICIPATED EXPENDITURES FOR NEXT YEAR

I.	Staff Salaries		$45,000
	Executive Director Ann McVee, M.S.W.	$11,500	
	Social Worker Sue Hill, B.S.W.	7,500	
	Rehabilitation Counselor Ron Bates, B.S.	6,600	
	Psychologist (one-half time) Jack Chappell, M.S.	6,000	
	Resident Manager (includes room and board) Ed Simms	3,000	
	Paraprofessional Worker Angie Wood	5,200	
	Secretary-Bookkeeper Mary Styles	5,200	
II.	Mortgage, insurance, and taxes on the house ($250 per month)		3,000
III.	Utilities ($150 per month)		1,800
IV.	Equipment, supplies (telephone, secretarial supplies, transportation, recreational needs, etc.)		5,000
V.	Food ($1.74 per person per day, for 23 persons*, for 365 days per year)		14,500
	TOTAL ANTICIPATED EXPENDITURES		$69,300

*Includes live-in resident manager

Bridge Place was the only place available to go for 12 of the current residents. Nine of the current residents had other options but still chose Bridge Place upon hospital release. Fifteen of the current residents are unmarried (either single, divorced, or separated). Most of the residents "like" Bridge Place, with 17 expressing satisfaction with the halfway house in general. It should be noted, however, that when asked about their preferences for an "ideal place to live," only 7 residents would choose the halfway house setting; 5 say they would like to live alone in an apartment, and 8 say they would like to share an apartment (either with or without ex-patients as apartment mates) where no staff are present.

Twelve of the current residents have paid jobs outside Bridge Place. Most of the remainder have "jobs" of some sort inside the halfway house (e.g., cleaning, washing dishes, helping to prepare meals, etc.), although a few are involved in community service projects away from the house (e.g., volunteer work at the Salvation Army or mental health association, etc.). David Thomas felt it was important that every resident have some type of regular work to be responsible for, as part of the transitional therapy from hospital back to community.

Residents' daily lives within Bridge Place are governed by a set of written rules compiled by staff, which include a requirement that residents "sign out" when leaving the house. Due to the recent downturn in the local economy (current unemployment rate is 9.5%), placements have become difficult and some residents who want to work are having trouble getting jobs. All but one of the current residents are white, 10 are male and 12 are female, the average age is 35, and the average educational level achieved is 13 years. Slightly less than half of the current residents are being supported (in toto or in part) by family, relatives, or social agencies. By diagnostic category, 14 have at one time been labeled as schizophrenics and 8 as nonpsychotic but with incapacitating neuroses. On the average, residents stay in Bridge Place between six and eight months.

The Staff

The staff at Bridge Place, like that at most psychiatric halfway houses, tend to be young--five of the six are under 40. Also, five of the staff are females, and all of the staff members are white. Compared to many other jobs, staff salaries at Bridge Place are low, and the work is demanding and intense. Thus, turnover has so far been quite high; only Sue Hill and Mary Styles were among the staff members present when Bridge Place was founded two years ago. Four of the current staff are married, while three are single, and one is divorced. Three of them have worked previously in a mental hospital in one capacity or another.

Dave Thomas, the original director who has just been replaced by Ann McVee, hired most of the present staff. He actually preferred "untrained" rather than trained staff because he felt that the requirements of the job in a halfway house do not involve doing therapy. Thus, he tended to select a mix of bachelor's degree and noncollege personnel. Ed Simms, the current house manager, is an older (age 37) undergraduate student, working on a B.S. degree in special education. He oversees the preparation of meals, supervises maintenance and clean-up, and is called on continuously by residents for support, ideas, and encouragement. Ed is well liked by both residents and staff and is considered to be an equal among all staff in all areas of decision making. This holds similarly for Angie Wood, a high school graduate, who works full time and who is in charge of recreational, social, and cultural activities for residents. Before leaving the agency, Dave Thomas wrote a memo to Ann McVee in which he briefly described the staff at Bridge Place (see Figure 2).

Most of the staff at Bridge Place like their jobs, due in part to the fact that the work setting is informal and they are free to innovate. There is currently, however, a 50-50 split among the staff over the issue of whether traditional psychotherapy should be offered. Traditional psychotherapy, in this instance, refers to one-to-one therapy which is both intensive and long term. Some of the staff feel that such therapy is very germane to successful rehabilitation and that brief counseling and occupational therapy are insufficient for helping the residents improve. Others feel just as strongly that the halfway

Figure 2

M E M O R A N D U M

TO: Ann McVee

FROM: David Thomas

RE: Current Staff at Bridge Place

     Before checking out, I thought it might be helpful to you if I left a brief description of my impressions of the Bridge Place staff. Since I had a hand in hiring most of them, it may help you to be aware of my assessments of their potential. Sorry I didn't get to see you before I left. Good luck!!

Mary Styles--Your bookkeeper and secretary--loyal, smart, and very good at what she does. She started half time when the program was launched and moved to full time a year later. She works 8 a.m. to 3 p.m. so she can be home when her children arrive from school. Angie or Ed or residents themselves cover the phone after she leaves. Her time is devoted totally to administration, though she is friendly and supportive toward residents at all times.

Angie Wood--One of the program's two paraprofessionals--a high school graduate who, after 12 years as a desk clerk at the Holiday Inn, decided to "work with people." She's had two years of experience as a teacher's aide and one year as a paraprofessional in the admissions ward of a private mental hospital in another state. She's a very capable person, cheerful and positive toward the residents and other staff--personally secure--willing to try new things. Her major assigned responsibility is the "social, recreational, and cultural" aspect of the program, although she regularly assists other staff in any number of activities on an "as-needed" basis.

Ed Simms--Resident manager--lives at Bridge Place 24 hours per day (with from Sunday noon to Monday evening off each week). A patient, conscientious, low-key person, he is highly regarded by the residents. His only experience in the human services has been as a ward attendant in a regional mental hospital. Working currently on his B.S. in special education, he hopes to go into the retardation field upon graduation. His salary is low ($250 month), but he receives free room and board plus free hospitalization insurance and free use of the van which belongs to the Bridge Place program. His duties include menu planning, shopping for food and supplies, organization and supervision of cooking, cleaning, and other housekeeping activities. Also, he provides constant support and assistance to the residents in all aspects of daily living.

Sue Hill--Bachelor's level social worker--one year of previous experience in a state mental hospital before joining the staff when Bridge Place was first opened. I hired her because I thought she had potential. She tends to take things quite literally and is somewhat resistant to changes or to new ideas. Her major duties include group and individual counseling of the residents around personal problems, interpersonal relations, family-related issues, etc. She would like to do therapy with the residents (as would Jack Chappell) and this was a sporadic source of contention between her and myself. Sue has perhaps been most effective in settling problems among residents over the refusal of some to do chores, to assume self-responsibility, etc.

Ron Bates--Like Sue Hill, a bachelor's level person--with a degree in rehabilitation services and six months experience in a state employment office. He knows his stuff in regard to vocational education, employment opportunities, and labor market trends. (He has not started to work as of this writing, but is scheduled to do so soon after I depart.) He seems enthusiastic and will improve with experience on the job and encouragement and support from you and his colleagues. I hired him because I hoped he would take the initiative in developing a job placement and follow-up plan for Bridge Place. Ron's predecessor (Larry Andrews) spent most of his time in one-to-one job counseling (regarding motivation, work habits, expectations) and was quite reluctant to interact with community resources on behalf of the residents.

Jack Chappell--Has a master's degree in community psychology and is working part time on a Ph.D. in counselor education--had three years' experience in the military as a psychological tester/evaluator. Jack came to us at the beginning of the second year of operation. Because of his age (he's 31) and experience (as compared to Sue and Ron), he plays a leadership role among the staff. Sometimes this is helpful and productive and sometimes it is not. Along with Sue, he would very much like to do intensive therapy with the residents. Jack comes in daily (except Saturdays) for four hours. On Monday and Thursday, he comes in from 8 a.m. to 12 noon, on Tuesday and Friday, from 1 to 5 p.m., and on Wednesday and Sunday, from 5 to 9 p.m. His hours are staggered so as to accommodate the variety of work and community-service schedules which characterize our residents. Jack's primary responsibility is psychological and aptitude testing and counseling as related to the interpretation and assessment of test results. Of course, he (like the rest of us) tries to be responsive to the great variety of requests for attention and time which our residents regularly make.

Dr. Matthew Zayles--Local psychiatrist who donates two hours of consultation time to Bridge Place each week. He tries to come in each Thursday from 8 to 10 a.m. Although he occasionally meets with a resident, his more typical pattern is to meet with the program staff and to offer suggestions regarding referrals (of our residents to other agencies), client drug dosages, etc. (I attended the staff meetings with Dr. Zayles on occasion, but was usually too involved with other matters to be able to do so.) He writes many of the prescriptions for our residents' chemotherapeutic needs, particularly for those who have no regular psychiatrist or other physician.

Dr. Freddie Carver--Donates medical services, on a call-basis only, to Bridge Place. During weekdays, we make every effort to get our residents to a private physician or to a clinic. However, on weekends, holidays, or in any emergency, Dr. Carver is very good about responding to our needs. Dr. Carver is one of the two physicians on our board of directors.

house setting is, in concept, incompatible with a traditional approach and that the welfare of the Bridge Place residents would be hindered rather than enhanced by employing this method. Further, they contend that the present staff lack expertise in this area. They feel that instead of attempting to use skills which they "don't have," they should instead capitalize on the ones they do have. It should be noted that Dave Thomas was quite adamant that traditional therapy not be offered. Ann McVee has not yet made her position clear.

On other issues, the staff are in greater consensus. For instance, two-thirds of them believe that it is important to provide structure for the residents in their daily activities (e.g., regular wake-up and bedtimes, regular meals, regular meetings, etc.) Also, fully 70% of the Bridge Place staff believe it is important to disperse client services among different agencies, rather than to try to provide all of them under one roof. In short, the present staff recognize the importance of strong ties with other agencies which can provide essential services for the Bridge Place residents.

Residents of Bridge Place feel positively toward the staff, but in many respects they are unclear about their expected relationships with staff members. Residents feel much more certain about what is expected of them vis-a-vis house rules and other residents than they do regarding resident-staff relations. In some ways, residents believe staff members expect greater conforming behavior from them than they should and tend to expect too little in the way of independence. It should be noted that during its two years of existence, there has not been any attention given to in-service training (or staff development) for the staff.

David Thomas

David Thomas, the original director, came to Bridge Place with a B.S. in finance, an M.S. in public administration, and no work experience as an administrator. He was a methodical and dedicated director, and people generally trusted him implicitly. His greatest interest, and perhaps expertise, lay in establishing a firm financial base under Bridge Place, assuring its survival as a new agency. In this respect, Dave showed great skill. However, some of the money which he secured has rather stiff conditions attached to it, and these conditions are about to result in pressures on Bridge Place to alter some of its program and commitments. Ann McVee is slowly becoming aware of these price tags, most of which were not identified during her interviews before accepting the job.

Dave spent almost all of his time and energy on matters outside the halfway house itself. Thus, the program which exists at Bridge Place developed in something of a haphazard manner and tends to reflect each individual staff member's predilections rather than any overall philosophy or orientation. Further, when Dave started out, he hired two full-time people (Sue Hill and Larry Andrews) and one part-time person (Mary Styles). There was so much excitement over the newness of everything that no one gave much thought to the decision-making process and/or lines of authority at Bridge Place. When the necessity arose, the three-person staff would usually huddle for 15 minutes or so and attempt to resolve the issue at hand. However, since Dave was often away from Bridge Place, and since no one was designated as "second in command," decisions were often made by default. Also, occasionally nothing was done when definite action was called for. This pattern of inactivity, or reluctance to make and act on decisions (due to confusion regarding one's authority to do so), is still characteristic of the staff at Bridge Place and promises to be a problem for Ann McVee in her new job.

A final aspect of Dave's inattention to intrahouse matters is that the staff are unclear regarding the goals and objectives of the Bridge Place program--both for the residents and for the community at large. Should they be treating the residents for their mental problems? Or, should they assume that the residents are normal (or near normal) people, primarily in need of friendship, support, and supportive services (e.g., assistance in finding a job, in locating a place to live, in reestablishing community ties, in finding needed social services in regular social agencies, etc.)? The staff are fairly evenly split over these issues, and unless some consensus is reached, the residents are bound to suffer from the contradictory messages which they are currently receiving from staff.

It should be noted that Dave Thomas quit the job of executive
director of Bridge Place in order to take a new job with the state
which paid a considerably higher salary. At the time he left--18
months after Bridge Place was founded--he was very much liked by the
board of directors, and, although the staff had some misgivings about
his leadership at Bridge Place per se, they too thought he was a very
friendly and talented person. Five months lapsed before the board was
able to replace Dave. His replacement, who has now been on the job one
month, is Ann McVee.

Ann McVee

Ann has a bachelor's degree in political science and a master's
degree in social work. Her specialty in her master's program was
social administration. However, after completing her degree, and
before taking the directorship of Bridge Place, she worked for three
years as a counselor in a multipurpose mental health clinic in a nearby
state. Thus, although she has more work experience than Dave did, she
too is entering her first job as an administrator. She is excited
about the possibilities which she envisions for Bridge Place, though
she is somewhat insecure about her abilities to raise funds for its
support. During her job interviews, however, she was assured by
several of the board members that the finances were in fine shape--
since Dave Thomas was so good in that area. Whether or not this was an
accurate statement should become clear during the upcoming year.

When the directorship of Bridge Place was offered to her, Ann
McVee decided to accept the job. In order to do so, she actually took
a small reduction in salary ($300). However, it was her first
chance to try out her skills as an administrator and she had many ideas
regarding program development and community relations which she was
eager to try out. Knowing that she would need the support both of the
board of directors and of the halfway house staff and residents if she
was to be successful in implementing her ideas, she has spent the first
month attempting to get to know these people and to establish good
rapport with them. Believing that she has been successful in these
endeavors, she is ready to launch some of her plans.

The Locality

Campbell is a medium-sized city with 85,000 residents and is the county seat of Dibbs County which has a total population of 150,000. Most of the residents at Bridge Place have historically come from Dibbs County, with the majority being former residents of Campbell itself. While Bridge Place has no official policy which eliminates noncounty residents, its ties with the local mental health association and clinic unofficially commit it to serve local residents first. With the recent trend of increasing state hospital discharges, pressures have mounted on Bridge Place to take more residents and to take residents who are older than 45 years of age. Dave Thomas, and the board, originally limited the age range of residents from 21 to 35, because they felt that greater success could be achieved with younger residents (whose length of hospitalization has, generally, been brief). The change to a range of 21 to 45 was taken last year in response to the state mental health division office, and pressures are mounting to widen the range to include even older persons. This is certainly an issue which the Bridge Place director and staff will have to come to grips with soon.

Pressures from another source are also increasing. The Mill Valley Mental Health Clinic which is in Dibbs County is in the process of developing an extensive community mental health program. The clinic has contributed $8,000 to the Bridge Place budget for the upcoming year, as part of this development plan. In return for its support, the clinic is hoping that Bridge Place will admit larger numbers of community referrals, thus avoiding hospitalization for greater numbers of local residents. The clinic has the strong and aggressive support of the Dibbs County Mental Health Association in this endeavor. Thus, Bridge Place is going to be expected to admit more local residents who have never been hospitalized.

Ann McVee, the new executive director, is clearly concerned about these pressures for greater admissions. She considers that the floor space of the house is already at the point of overcrowding. While there are currently no accreditation standards for psychiatric halfway houses, she feels (as do other directors with whom she has talked) that it is vital for resident well-being that the halfway house setting not be overcrowded. Further, while it has not been done up to now,

Ms. McVee would like to revamp the programmatic format of Bridge Place so as to make it possible for social work, psychology, and rehabilitation student interns to have placements there and this would have a bearing on space usage and availability.

The problem of referral pressures is currently being aggravated by the recent difficulty of Bridge Place residents in finding full-time jobs. With employment opportunities limited, the residents are less able to move quickly to independent living, and the average length of stay has been slowly rising. During its two years of existence, Bridge Place has not had a bona fide placement program to help its residents find jobs. Dave Thomas was too busy raising money for the house's budget to worry about this aspect of the program. Larry Andrews, the first rehabilitation counselor, stayed at Bridge Place just over a year (and his position has only recently been filled by Ron Bates); during that first year, so much was happening as the program got underway that he did not have time to develop a placement program. And, while Sue Hill has worried about it, she really does not feel qualified to take the initiative in this area.

As a result of no explicit placement program, residents have generally looked for, applied for, and landed jobs on their own. While the economy was booming this worked out quite well. But with the current slump, such an approach is not working. The residents are becoming somewhat bitter because (as noted earlier) most of them would prefer to be on their own.

Neither Dave Thomas nor Ann McVee considers it necessary, nor even desirable, that all residents be placed in paid employment. Some may never be able to support themselves. However, residents generally prefer to be on their own, in some respect, and to play a useful role in society. Further, it is important for morale purposes that residents not be "stuck" in Bridge Place too long. Thus, Ann McVee feels that some creative thinking is called for regarding resident placements for the future.

Bridge Place has never done systematic follow-up on its former residents. Unless they have returned to the halfway house (either as residents or as visitors), the staff have no idea how well they are doing, where they are, whether they have been able to sustain

Figure 3

ANTICIPATED REVENUES FOR NEXT YEAR

Residents' weekly room/board payments
($37.50 per week x 22 residents x 52
weeks, less 15% for house less than
full, people unable to pay, etc.) $36,465

United Fund $ 6,000

Dibbs County Mental Health Association $ 2,000

Mill Valley Mental Health Clinic $ 8,000

Research and Demonstration Grant from
State Department of Mental Health ($15,000/
year for two years; second year just
beginning) $15,000

TOTAL ANTICIPATED REVENUES $67,465

Note: Anticipated revenues of $67,465 are less (approximately $2,000)
than anticipated expenses of $69,300.

independent living, etc. The research and demonstration grant which
Dave Thomas secured from the state entails a commitment by Bridge Place
to evaluate the long-term effects of its program. However, since Dave
quit his job as executive director within six months after the grant
was awarded, nothing was ever done about this aspect of it. Ann McVee,
who has now been on the job one month, knows that this is something to
which she and her staff must give attention soon. (See Figure 3.)

Community Relations

A recurring issue for the Bridge Place program is its relationship
to the community. That is, exactly what is Bridge Place's obligation
to the community? Like most independent halfway houses, Bridge Place
is quite dependent on strong community ties and support. Thus, since
Dave Thomas was fearful of antagonizing community leaders and agency
personnel, he tended to promise a positive response--though, often,
only implicitly--to whatever requests they made of Bridge Place.
Either he apparently felt that such requests would be relatively easy
to fulfill or else he simply did not think about them much. At any
rate, his fear of jeopardizing community ties may have played a role in
the development of the fairly tight staff controls over residents which
characterizes Bridge Place currently. Dave may have felt that the
house simply could not run the risk of unfavorable publicity due to
unpredictable resident activities or behavior.

In this connection, a crucial aspect of Bridge Place's
relationship to the neighborhood in which it exists should be noted.
Like approximately three-fourths of all psychiatric halfway houses,
Bridge Place remains anonymous to its immediate neighborhood. That is,
except for its official agency and community liaisons, it does not
engage in or encourage interaction with neighbors, nor does it seek

publicity on a community-wide level.* Dave Thomas's rationale for this involved two points: (1) anonymity reduces the chances of confrontations with neighbors who might be upset by its location in their neighborhood; and (2) anonymity reduces the likelihood of further labeling of Bridge Place residents as "mental patients." The second point was, in fact, used by Dave on occasion to justify the house's lack of a fully developed job- and housing-placement program for residents. He felt that the residents of Bridge Place would run less risk of additional stigmatization if they sought jobs and housing on their own, with little or no official help from the Bridge Place staff. Whether this is a valid rationalization is not at all clear.

---

*Organizations seeking to establish a halfway house have to deal with local governmental officials in order to comply with zoning requirements and/or restrictions in locating the house. Once the house is established, furthermore, liaisons and linkages are generally established with other agencies and organizations to and from which halfway house clients are referred. Our point is that, in the general case, contact with the local community has generally been restricted to relevant governmental and human service agencies.

FRAME I

RELATIONSHIP OF BRIDGE PLACE TO OTHER AGENCIES

ORIENTATION

Ann McVee has been executive director of Bridge Place for one month. She is now faced with a crisis that affects not only Bridge Place's relationships with other agencies (on whom they must depend to provide services to their residents) but also the financial foundation of Bridge Place itself. Dr. Atwood, director of the Mill Valley Mental Health Clinic, and Ms. Harroff, executive director of the Dibbs County Mental Health Association, have written to Ms. McVee, charging that Bridge Place has not fulfilled its promises to either agency (i.e., Bridge Place has failed to accept persons into the halfway house before they are hospitalized in an effort to prevent hospitalization). Both agencies are threatening to cut off the funds which they have contributed to Bridge Place in the past if this situation is not remedied.

Step 1. Setting the Scene (5 minutes)

Note to Participants: Divide now into groups of six. You will be working with this group throughout the entire simulation. The roles which each of you assume may vary, but you will be working with the same people. The purpose of this continuity of group membership is to simulate the environment of a real agency where you work with the same people to solve different problems.

Each of you should read the memo written by Dr. Atwood and Ms. Harroff to Ann McVee which appears in Figure 4. Review the budget documents which are in the Background Frame (Figures 1 and 3). When all of you have read this material, proceed to the next step.

Figure 4

M E M O R A N D U M

TO: Ms. Ann McVee, Executive Director of Bridge Place

FROM: Dr. Atwood, Director of Mill Valley Mental Health Clinic
        Ms. Harroff, Executive Director, Dibbs County Mental Health
        Association

RE: Referrals from the Mill Valley Clinic to Bridge Place

You have been in the position of executive director at Bridge Place now for one month. Our association with you has, thus far, been quite pleasant and we have every confidence that you are a highly talented person. However, we are gravely concerned about certain aspects of the Bridge Place program, and we feel it only fair to apprise you of our position before we take further action.

As you know, between the two organizations which we represent (the Mill Valley Clinic and the Dibbs County Mental Health Association), a total of $10,000 was given to Bridge Place to use as needed to support your program during the present fiscal year. To our knowledge, this represents almost 15% of your current annual budget, and thus cannot be considered an insignificant sum. Our hopes--indeed, our expressed objectives--upon giving this money to Bridge Place were that your facility would serve, to an ever increasing extent, those of our local residents who have emotional problems which are serious but not severe. That is, we expected to be able to refer many of our moderately disturbed patients to you, thereby avoiding the necessity of their institutionalization at one of our state hospitals. The savings in human misery and heartbreak which this service to the local area would represent are inestimable. In this respect, your program has been a grave disappointment to us. To corroborate our point, Ms. Harroff's administrative assistant has done some research and discovered that of the 17 persons whom the clinic has referred to Bridge Place in the past two and one-half years, your halfway house has accepted a total of 2.

We realize that most of our discussions around this issue were conducted not with you, but with your predecessor, Mr. David Thomas. Thus, perhaps you have been less than fully aware of the reciprocal commitments between our respective organizations. Also, we acknowledge that we are perhaps at fault for not putting this agreement in writing. We believe that Mr. Thomas had full understanding of Bridge Place's side of the bargain, however, and we, in good faith, expected the agreement to be complied with. Certainly, we have kept our part of the bargain by transferring the promised funds to your program.

Both of our organizations are currently in the process of budget negotiations for the upcoming fiscal year. Based on your record of nonresponsiveness to us to date, we feel extremely reluctant to ask our boards to continue to support your program.

We suggest that you and your board give serious consideration to a drastic revision of your admissions policies. We hope that you will give highest priority to referrals from the Mill Valley Clinic who are in need of your program's services. We certainly feel that some reciprocation on your part is called for. We shall be happy to meet with you and your board over this issue.

Step 2. What Is the Problem? (15 minutes)

You are free to organize your group of six in any way you see fit to accomplish the task at hand. Your entire group will be defining a problem from the perspective of Ann McVee's administrative role of executive director of Bridge Place. Although Ann McVee is one person, she fulfills at least three functions:

--Fiscal Manager. This part of Ann McVee is concerned about the financial stability of Bridge Place and realizes that it is in danger of losing 15% of its annual budget. The board of directors is usually very concerned about fiscal matters.

--Supervisor of Bridge Place. This part of Ann McVee is concerned about changes being pushed by Atwood and Harroff, which, if implemented, would have dramatic impact upon staff functioning and morale. She is also concerned about the residents at Bridge Place and wonders how the potential influx of new types of residents will affect their interrelationships.

--Community Relations Specialist. This part of Ann McVee is concerned about Bridge Place's relationships with the community and community agencies, and she knows that her handling of this crisis can make or break her with the community.

In this step, you need to define the problem. Again, you are free to organize yourselves in any manner you prefer in order to complete this task. While trying to define the problem posed by the Atwood-Harroff memo, you might wish to be guided by the following questions:

1. Exactly what is it that Atwood and Harroff want Bridge Place to do?

2. If Bridge Place complies with their demands, how will Bridge Place be affected over the next six months? Over the next two years?

3. If Bridge Place refuses to meet their demands, how will Bridge Place be affected over the next six months? Over the next two years?

<u>Step 3. Developing a Solution</u> (30 minutes)

There are many ways to go about solving a problem. One way is to follow "whatever feels right." Another way which has been successful is to identify clearly the criteria by which you would choose which solution is a "good" solution, to brainstorm, to think of all the possible solutions without analyzing them, and to apply the criteria you have developed to the list of possible solutions in order to choose the "best" solution. Criteria that could be used in attempting to develop a solution to the Atwood-Harroff dilemma include the following:

1. The value Ann McVee places on her reputation as an administrator.

2. The value placed on retaining the Bridge Place program as it is currently operating.

3. The value placed on good working relationships with agencies such as the Mill Valley Mental Health Clinic and the Dibbs County Mental Health Association.

4. The impact of any solution (short and/or long range) on staff and residents.

Work now within your group to develop a solution to the problem facing Bridge Place. When you feel you have reached a good solution, check to make certain you have stated who does what, when, and with whom. Include also the major strength and major weakness of your proposed solution.

When your group has finished this step, wait for your instructor before proceeding to the next step.

Step 4. Debriefing (25 minutes)

1. Each group of six should make a brief presentation to the other groups. State criteria used, the solution, and how the solution reflects the criteria. Include also the major strength and weakness of your proposed solution.

2. Recall the three major functions of Ann McVee (fiscal manager, supervisor of Bridge Place, and community relations specialist). In developing your own group's solution, which functional part of Ann McVee was the strongest? Do you think this is true in real life?

3. To what extent was Bridge Place at fault in this situation? What could/should be done in the future to prevent such problems from occurring again?

4. Why do you think organizations resist putting agreements in writing?

FRAME II

PRIORITIZING ISSUES AND TASK FORCE PLANNING

ORIENTATION

Bridge Place has regular, weekly staff meetings. The primary agenda item for the next meeting will be Ann McVee's memorandum to the staff regarding the goals of Bridge Place (see Figure 5). As staff, your assigned task is: (1) to address the questions raised in McVee's memorandum; (2) to identify those aspects of the Bridge Place situation and program which need attention; (3) to prioritize the issues in terms of immediacy and overall importance to the survival of Bridge Place; and (4) to develop plans to implement resolution of these issues.

Step 1. Getting Ready (5 minutes)

Within your group, each participant should choose a number between 1 and 6. Numbers may not be chosen twice. Depending upon which number you chose, you will play the role of the following person in the upcoming staff meeting (and throughout Frame II and Frame III):
  1. Ron Bates;
  2. Angie Wood;
  3. Jack Chappell;
  4. Ann McVee;
  5. Ed Simms;
  6. Sue Hill.

Turn again to the Background Frame to reread Figure 2 (the memo from Dave Thomas to Ann McVee concerning staff) in order to understand the role you are about to play. The person who is playing the role of Ann McVee should review the special section under "Staff" in the Background Frame. Ann McVee must remember that she always has at least three concerns: (1) the residents and staff of Bridge Place; (2) the board of directors of Bridge Place; and (3) the community (including other mental health agencies, employers, the public at large, the neighborhood in which Bridge Place is located, and so forth).

When each of you has read his/her role description and Figure 5 (which appears on the following page), proceed to the next step.

Figure 5

M E M O R A N D U M

TO: The Staff of Bridge Place

FROM: Ann McVee, Director

RE: Questions Related to Our Program's
        Future: Needs and Goals

        Getting to know you over the past month has been a pleasant and
rewarding experience. I am looking forward to working with each of you
on the many aspects of our excellent, but developing, program here at
Bridge Place. Having just returned from a Region VI Conference for
directors of community-based mental health programs, I would like to
share with you some things which I learned there. Also, I would like
to pose a number of questions about our program's future direction.
These are, I believe, of concern both to you and to myself.

        A major theme of the conference was the constant reminder to us
that the halfway house is a transitional facility. As one halfway
house director put it, "The halfway house can aid a former mental
patient's tenuous transition into the community by providing a
residential facility that affords an informal, warm and supportive
milieu" (Gumrucku, 1968). This director went on to remind us that
since the halfway house concept commits us to resident reentry and
reintegration into the community, each halfway house program must
establish and maintain strong community ties.

        With these points in mind, I pose a number of questions for your
consideration. In preparation for next Tuesday's staff meeting, I hope
you will give serious thought to each of them. Please come to the
meeting (at 2 p.m.) with your ideas and suggestions.

    1. In your opinion, what are the greatest strengths of our
        Bridge Place program? On what do you base your judgments?

    2. In your opinion, what are the greatest weaknesses of our
        program? What are your reasons for saying this?

    3. What things need our attention most urgently?

    4. What things need to be carefully thought out and planned
        before action is taken?

    5. What would you like to see changed about our program:
        either added and/or deleted?

    6. How would you most like to be involved in the program here
        at Bridge Place? (i.e., doing what types of things? for
        whom? when? how? where?)

Step 2. Wrestling with the Issues (20 minutes)

The first step in the staff meeting is to determine the list of issues which you, the staff, must face. Based upon your knowledge of Bridge Place and Ann McVee's memorandum to staff, read the list of issues which appears on the following page. If there are other issues which are not included in this list, please add them to the bottom of the list. If there are issues included in the list which you feel are not relevant or are not truly issues, feel free to delete them from the list. A majority of staff members must agree to the addition or deletion of any issue from the list.

After deciding on the issues to be included, rank and weight each issue according to the following instructions. If you are not unanimous, a majority vote will establish priorities. In case of a tie, Ann McVee will make a decision for the entire staff.

1. Rank order the issues in terms of the urgency which you, the Bridge Place staff, feel the issue deserves. Rank as "1" the issue which you feel must receive the most immediate attention; "2" as the issue which is second in immediacy; and so on. Tied ranks are not allowed.

2. Assign a percentage of time to each issue which you have ranked. This percentage will represent the amount of attention which the staff, as a whole, should give to the issue over the next six months. In a way, these percentages will reflect the importance of an issue to Bridge Place's functioning and survival and not necessarily its urgency.

LIST OF ISSUES

Rank   % of Time

_____ A. Development and implementation of a job/housing placement program for residents. _____

_____ B. Devise and implement a follow-up procedure for determining the status of past residents and of future "discharges." _____

_____ C. Clarification of lines of authority and decision-making procedures; clarification of roles and responsibilities of staff members and of residents. _____

_____ D. Focusing the treatment program of Bridge Place and clarifying the goals and objectives of the halfway house program; clarification of the purpose and modes of in-house vs. outside service provision, etc. _____

_____ E. Clarification and articulation of goals and objectives of Bridge Place vis-a-vis the community (e.g., what are its obligations: to other agencies in general? to agencies which provide financial support? to citizens in the local area? to mental patients in general? to the state mental health program? etc.). _____

_____ F. Addressing financial problems and goals (e.g., how to raise additional funds to meet current year's expenses; seeking new sources of support; deletion of staff due to financial problems; etc.). _____

_____ G. _____

_____

_____ _____
(additional issue)

_____ H. _____

_____

_____ _____
(additional issue)

Step 3. Task Force Planning for Implementation (30 minutes)

Assume that one week has passed since the last staff meeting. You are now to organize yourselves into the two task forces to plan for the implementation of the priorities which were established in the last step. Divide into two task forces, Task Force 1 and Task Force 2. Task Force 1 will work on the issue that received first priority in the last step. Task Force 2 will work on the issue that received second priority.

In developing your plans for implementation, you may find it helpful to work through the questions that appear on the following page. As you plan for the future Bridge Place program, remember three things: (1) you will need to convince your fellow staff that your plan is worthy of implementation; (2) you will need to live with the results of your plan, if and when it is implemented; and (3) the survival of Bridge Place may depend on the ability of you and your fellow staff members to implement the plans you propose.

ISSUE: _____

1. Why is this a priority issue?

2. What objectives should be met in resolving this issue?

3. What strategies (who, when, and how) should be used?

4. What programs should therefore be developed? (Include operational details.)

FRAME III

DECISION MAKING IN THE CONTEXT OF DAILY PRESSURES

ORIENTATION

Continue to play the role which you played in Frame II. Consider that you are once again assembled as the full programmatic staff of Bridge Place, that a regular staff meeting is about to take place, and that Ann McVee will chair the meeting. It is now six weeks after the Tuesday staff meeting in which Ann McVee's memo was first discussed. The major agenda item for this staff meeting is that each of the Task Forces will report to the full staff on the plans which it has developed and an attempt will be made to decide which plans to implement.

Step 1. Presenting Suggestions (15 minutes)

With Ann McVee chairing the meeting, moving it along to make certain that each Task Force is allowed equal time to present its suggestions, the staff of Bridge Place will meet to listen to each Task Force's suggestions (as they were developed in the prior frame). Name the issue with which you were working and then outline the programs, goals, strategies, operational details, and (if necessary) your rationale. Move quickly, as you will want to make certain both Task Forces have a chance to speak. Do not discuss or debate the merits of any of the suggestions; use this time to acquaint all members of the staff with the various Task Forces' work.

Write the suggestions of the Task Force of which you were not a member on the following page.

ISSUE: _____

1. Why is this a priority issue?

2. What goals should be met in resolving this issue?

3. What strategies (who, when, and how) should be used?

4. What programs should therefore be developed? (Include operational details.)

Step 2. Dealing with Daily Pressures (30 minutes)

Ann McVee had planned to continue the staff meeting after the Task Force presentations had been made so that the staff as a whole could decide which aspects of each plan to accept and/or reject. The phone rings three times in quick succession, however, and the following messages are relayed to the staff by McVee after she finishes each conversation:

> --One of your residents called from the police station.
> Phil Lakeman has been arrested for theft, and he's using
> his one phone call to reach Bridge Place. He does not have
> sufficient cash with him to post bail, nor does he know the
> name of an attorney.

> --Jay Silverman, another resident, has gone home for three
> days as an experiment. The wife of the resident calls,
> saying that he's locked himself in the bedroom and won't
> respond to her calling him or knocking on the door. Other
> than calling the rescue squad or an ambulance, she doesn't
> know what to do.

> --The hospital called. Annie Campbell has been seriously hurt
> and is unconscious. McVee was unable to determine if she
> was in an accident or tried to commit suicide.

What will you, as staff, do now? Will you assign some of your members to act on some of these problems immediately? If so, which ones? Can some of them wait until the conclusion of the meeting? If so, which ones? What is going to happen to your plans devised by each Task Force?

Spend the next 30 minutes resolving these problems.

Step 3. Debriefing (30 minutes)

The questions below relate to Frames II and III which you just completed.

1. What did you do to cope with the residents' crises in the last frame? Who decided what would be done? What is the role of a supervisor in such a situation?

2. How can a halfway house balance the need to deal with everyday problems with the need to plan for the future?

3. How realistic are the tasks which you decided upon for the Bridge Place staff to achieve? In real life, could they achieve them? Which ones are the least realistic? The most realistic? Why?

4. How effectively did your Task Force go about fulfilling its charge? Did you have enough information to plan effectively? What was most frustrating about your charge? Most rewarding?

5. How did Ann McVee perform in the role of executive director? What did she do best? What could/should she have done differently?

6. Which aspects, if any, of the Bridge Place program should Ann McVee have planned for in Frame II (i.e., either by herself and/or in conjunction with her board of directors)? In short, was it inappropriate to have the staff involved in all aspects of planning/goal setting? Are any negative consequences or effects likely to result from this?

FRAME IV

RELATIONSHIP OF BRIDGE PLACE TO THE PUBLIC

ORIENTATION

No sooner has the staff set its program priorities than another crisis arises. Citizens in the local neighborhood where Bridge Place is located have discovered that Bridge Place houses "crazy people" and they are outraged (see Figure 6 on the next page). In fact, they are vowing to have Bridge Place moved from the neighborhood. In recent years, psychiatric halfway houses have learned--through hard experience--that over the long run it is unwise to locate in neighborhoods without local involvement. However, as noted in the Background Frame, Bridge Place chose to remain anonymous to its neighbors.

At this point, the chief spokesman for the neighborhood group, Mr. Dubose, has already met with Ms. McVee regarding his concerns. Also, he has met with the Executive Committee of the Bridge Place board of directors. In short, it is now clear to everyone involved that Mr. Dubose and his associates are very serious. Everyone who favors the continuation of Bridge Place as a mental health facility is gravely concerned about its future.

Figure 6

_____

NEWS RELEASE

City of Campbell (Dibbs County)

Citizens in the Parkside neighborhood of northwest Campbell held an emotion-ladened neighborhood meeting last night regarding the presence of a psychiatric halfway house, Bridge Place, in their section of town. They complained that the halfway house was "secretly and furtively" located in their neighborhood, and that they were given no opportunity to express their feelings about its location there.

One local resident, Mr. J. C. Dubose, was elected spokesman for the group. In an interview, he said that the neighborhood residents were appalled at the idea of having a bunch of "lunatics" living in the same area where they are trying to raise children. The neighborhood, he went on to say, "is in danger of urban deterioration, anyway. And we fear that something like this may be the straw that breaks the camel's back. All we need now is for the younger families to begin a mass exodus from the area."

The group is considering a number of alternative actions aimed at the removal of Bridge Place from their neighborhood. "If we have to take them to court, we will," said one man. Other options include a request to the City Council's Zoning Commission to rule on the legality of such a facility in a residential area. Also, Mr. Dubose says he plans to meet with the director of Bridge Place, Ms. Ann McVee, in the next day or so. He is hopeful that she will understand the position which he represents and will agree to voluntarily move Bridge Place to another section of town. He reiterated that he has nothing against the halfway house concept in general, but that he is adamantly opposed to the location of such facilities in neighborhoods where there are children.

_____

Step 1. Reaction of the Executive Director (20 minutes)

You must cope with your outraged neighbors. All of you should collectively play the role of Ann McVee, executive director of Bridge Place. The Executive Committee of the Bridge Place board of directors has charged Ann McVee with devising a strategy for resolving the current crisis. Specifically, they have asked her to present to the board the following: (1) a range of alternative actions which could be taken in response to the present situation; (2) a recommendation (and rationale) for one or more preferred alternatives; (3) a plan for accomplishing the preferred alternatives; and (4) a long-range strategy for avoiding such unfavorable events and publicity in the future.

Since all of you will play the role of Ann McVee, you are free to organize yourselves in any way you see fit. One person should be designated as recorder so that all plans and recommendations will be recorded for the time when Ann McVee reports back to the Bridge Place board.

I.   Alternatives

II.   Recommendation and Rationale

III. Specific Plan

IV.   Long-Range Strategy

Step 2. Reaction of the Board (30 minutes)

Due to your work in the last step, Ann McVee now has a strategy worked out to deal with the neighborhood. In this step, she will present that strategy to the board, and the board and she will work together to find a way to meet the threat posed to Bridge Place by its neighbors.

Within your group, assign one member to each of the following roles:

1. Ann McVee;
2. Abraham (Abe) Cohen;
3. Mary Lou Harroff;
4. Freddie Carver;
5. Sam Proctor;
6. Susan Mabe.

Turn to the following pages to read the role description which has been assigned to you. Read your role description only.

When each of you has finished reading his/her role description, begin the role play. First, each member should introduce him/herself as the character he/she is to play and give his/her position within the community and on the board. Then Ann McVee will outline her suggested strategy (from Step 1) to cope with the crisis created by Bridge Place's neighbors. After McVee is through speaking, Mr. Cohen (the board chairman) will proceed with the meeting in any way he sees fit. The goal is to come up with a good plan to solve the crisis created by the neighborhood uproar over Bridge Place.

Role Description for <u>Ann McVee</u>, Executive Director of Bridge Place

Your job is to represent the Bridge Place program, residents, staff, philosophy, goals, and so forth. You are quite concerned about the most recent crisis, and you wonder if they're ever going to stop. You are uneasy about Ms. Harroff being here today. She has jumped on you before, with the hassle over Bridge Place's accepting more prehospitalization patients (Frame I). You will treat her very gingerly, with the utmost tact. As director of the Dibbs County Mental Health Association, she is in a position (perhaps more so than any other board member) to help or harm Bridge Place.

Outline your strategy (which you developed in the last step) carefully to the Executive Committee of the board. Be sure to point out its strengths and potential weaknesses.

Role Description for <u>Abraham (Abe) Cohen</u>, Chairman of the Bridge Place
    Board of Directors

You are a practicing clinical psychologist in Campbell and
chairman of the board of directors of Bridge Place. You know that the
board of directors is legally responsible for everything that happens
at Bridge Place. This means that you can be personally liable, should
the neighbors really get organized and take their complaint to court.

You're interested in solving this problem quickly and, most of
all, permanently. It is important to you that all members of the
Executive Committee have a chance to speak. You like to balance all
viewpoints, believing that it leads to a good end product.

Role Description for <u>Mary Lou Harroff</u>, Board Member

You are a member of the board of directors for Bridge Place and the executive director of the Dibbs County Mental Health Association. You are still upset about the composition of Bridge Place's residents; you brought this issue up when McVee had been at Bridge Place for an entire month and had not taken any action. You feel that the neighbors would not be nearly as upset if most of the residents at Bridge Place were people who had not been hospitalized.

Your position with the local mental health association makes you the one member of the board who is in the greatest position of influence, relative to the community. You can agree to throw the entire association behind Bridge Place, backing them up and probably easing them out of this tight spot. Or you can remain silent, claiming you have no authority to commit the association to either side of such a controversial issue, and thus hurt Bridge Place.

Which position you take today depends a great deal upon how McVee presents herself and her ideas, and how she relates to you during the meeting. At some point during the meeting, you will announce your intentions regarding the mental health association's active support or nonsupport of Bridge Place during this crisis.

Remember that you were initially very enthusiastic about Bridge Place, but their continuing policy of accepting posthospitalization patients has been a great disappointment to you.

Role Description for <u>Freddie Carver</u>, Board Member

You are a member of the board of directors for Bridge Place. In addition, you serve the halfway house as an "on call" physician. You feel that the program at Bridge Place is in excellent shape, and you are quite angry toward the neighbors who wish to ruin this terrific program. You're not certain that you know exactly what to do about it, but you do know that you're angry and that you want to squelch this controversy as quickly and as completely as possible.

Defending Ann McVee is also important to you. You feel that she has done a good job. You also know that she and the previous director have very different administrative styles and thus, comparisons between the two are unfair.

Role Description for <u>Sam Proctor</u>, Board Member

You are a member of the board of directors of Bridge Place and a successful real estate broker. You represent the "businessman's orientation" on the board. Accordingly, you feel that the first thing any agency must do is <u>to survive</u>. If survival means moving Bridge Place then, for heaven's sake, move it. Principles of who is right and who is wrong are not as important as the survival of the halfway house.

You feel that if the residents presented a better image to the neighborhood, the neighbors wouldn't be upset. In your mind, "presenting a better image" means being employed in a full-time job. Many of the residents don't hold such jobs. You feel that if they did, no one would have room to complain because the residents would prove themselves to be hard-working, normal people. You will bring up the issue of full-time jobs for residents.

Although you and Ann McVee don't always agree on every point, you certainly wish to support her. You feel she needs at least a year to become totally acquainted with her job, and you want to give her every opportunity to succeed as well as Dave Thomas succeeded.

Role Description for <u>Susan Mabe</u>, Board Member

You are a member of the board of directors for Bridge Place. You are the assistant city manager of Campbell and a social worker. As such, you know that Bridge Place is a unique and needed part of the community. You are equally aware what a grave threat the neighborhood poses to Bridge Place.

The Dibbs County Mental Health Association can help Bridge Place a great deal--probably more than any other single individual or agency. Mary Lou Harroff, who is executive director of the association, sits on the board. You will push her to make a strong commitment on behalf of her association to help Bridge Place out of this tight bind. You feel that if her association conducted an intensive educational and public relations campaign in Campbell, with particular attention focused on Bridge Place's immediate neighborhood, the current crisis could be abated almost overnight.

Ms. Harroff might bring up the issue of prehospitalization residents for Bridge Place again (as she did in Frame I). If she does, you will become angry with her. You feel that her bringing that issue up when Ann McVee had been here only one month was unfair. Although you haven't done so yet, you'd really like to tell her that <u>that</u> one (particularly the threat of cutting off funds) was a blow below the belt. Today might be the day you do that.

Step 3. Debriefing (10 minutes)

1. If the board meeting had continued, what do you think would have been the eventual outcome? Why?

2. Given Dave Thomas's reasons for having Bridge Place remain anonymous in the neighborhood when it was founded, do you think this was the right thing to do? Why?

3. In the event one decided to seek neighborhood acceptance before locating a psychiatric halfway house, what (in your opinion) would be its chances for receiving such neighborhood support?

FRAME V

CHANGING THE PROGRAM

ORIENTATION

Two months have passed since the group of neighborhood citizens headed by Mr. Dubose confronted Bridge Place with their desire to rid their neighborhood of the Bridge Place halfway house. After careful consideration, the board decided (with McVee's complete concurrence) to resist the pressure to move Bridge Place. The citizens' group, therefore, decided to take their case for removal to the courts, where it is now in process.

The board members' decision to resist local ejection efforts stems from three points: (1) they believe that the objections to the location of Bridge Place in the neighborhood are incorrect and ill-founded; (2) they know that the location of Bridge Place is in compliance with local zoning laws; and (3) they believe it would be disruptive to the residents and to the program to change locations at this time. Board members have agreed, however, that if either of the following situations ensues, they will plan for a future relocation of the facility: (a) if Bridge Place loses the case in the lower courts, they will not appeal and will move; or (b) even if Bridge Place wins the case in court, unless local sentiment can be either ameliorated or changed, they will eventually move.

Using a $1,000 cash gift to Bridge Place by a local patron, McVee recently hired two consultants for the Bridge Place program. They come in one at a time to run workshops of 1½ days each to provide in-service training for the Bridge Place staff. Each consultant had previously worked in and conducted research on psychiatric halfway houses. McVee, along with some of her staff, were very impressed with the consultants' observations and advice. (A summary of their recommendations appears in Figure 7.)

As the executive director, McVee is now in the position of having to decide whether she will attempt to convince the Bridge Place board, as well as some members of her own staff, that program changes in line with the consultants' suggestions are advisable. In reaching her decision, one factor which she must consider is Sue Hill's threat to quit the Bridge Place program if such changes are implemented. Although Hill claims that her reasons for leaving would be the program changes, McVee suspects that Sue may be looking for an excuse to leave Bridge Place. McVee's major worry is that Hill will become disgruntled and, upon leaving, will complain to the press about the "crazy new program" at Bridge Place.

If McVee decides not to institute the changes, she will have to do something about staff and resident morale. Ever since the neighborhood citizens' protest and the negative news coverage, staff and residents have felt very low and discouraged. This is one reason McVee decided to use the gift of $1,000 to hire program consultants. She felt that both she and the staff needed a "shot in the arm."

Step 1. Devising Plans (20 minutes)

As you have done previously in this simulation, all of you will collectively play the role of Ann McVee. You are free to organize yourselves within your group of six in any way you see fit. A summation of the consultants' suggestions appears on the following page. They are taken from McVee's notes during the time the consultants spent at Bridge Place. Read them before you do anything else.

After you have read her notes, decide among yourselves what course McVee will pursue. Should she be cautious and simply try to keep Bridge Place in a "holding status" until the location program is settled? Since legal actions often drag on for months, this may be a frustrating course of nonaction. On the other hand, should McVee attempt to implement the program changes and run the risk of unanticipated problems, stresses, and strains which they may entail? Once you make a decision regarding which course to pursue, develop written justifications for the following items on the next page:

1. Develop a rationale for your decision for use in gaining board support for it.

2. Develop a strategy to gain staff and resident cooperation and support for your decision (including a contingency plan in the event Sue Hill leaves Bridge Place in a disgruntled state).

Figure 7

NOTES ON THE CONSULTANTS' VISITS

Both consultants had a great deal of useful information and advice to impart to staff. They reported, for example, that halfway houses with the best success rates (of permanent community placements) are those which have high expectations of residents combined with high demands for performance. This means, in general, that residents should be expected to be responsible for themselves. That is, staff should insist on resident self-sufficiency. For example, residents should be expected to plan and prepare their own meals, clean their own rooms, do their own laundry, establish their own rules (as a group) and enforce them, and so on. Staff play an important role in establishing a climate in which standards for resident functioning can emerge. Staff can also reinforce residents when they behave independently and self-sufficiently. In short, staff should serve more as reinforcers and as resource persons rather than as guardians, caretakers, or overseers. Services provided to residents by the halfway house staff should focus on relevant personal, social, and occupational behaviors which will assist in the reestablishing of independent community living.

Among the consultants' criticisms of the present Bridge Place program were the observations that: (1) the staff take too much responsibility for the residents; (2) the staff need to have higher expectations regarding what residents can and should do; and (3) the Bridge Place program needs to be more demanding of its residents. Even those residents who, for example, are unable to gain or maintain outside employment should be required to work a certain number of hours per day. This could include tasks in the halfway house (such as meal preparation, filing, housecleaning) or volunteer work in a community agency.

The consultants praised the program for restricting its resident population to around 20 or so clients, cautioning that a larger number of clients tends to result in less successful client outcomes. Additionally, the fact that staff members perform a variety of duties and roles is considered to be a plus. The consultants noted that when staff perform a number of specialized but complementary roles, clients tend to fare better upon discharge. Reasons for this include higher rates of staff-to-staff interaction required for coordination when roles and duties are distinct. Finally, the program was praised for its "good" staff/client ratio (i.e., the number of nonclerical staff divided by the number of clients). A ratio of .27 (or 6 divided by 22) means that there is one staff member for about every four clients. A higher staff/client ratio is typically associated with higher success rates after discharge for clients of residential treatment facilities.

3. Devise a strategy for actually: (a) implementing the program changes, if any; (b) for boosting staff and resident morale.

In the event you decide to attempt the program changes, give some attention to each of these questions: What "supports" will you provide for staff who may become insecure (threatened or defensive) as the residents become less dependent on them? How will you prepare both residents and staff for the disorder and disarray which will likely characterize the initial stages of the change? How long do you anticipate it will be before the positive results or benefits of the change begin to emerge?

Designate one member of your group to record decisions and plans so that McVee can report to the board (and so your group can report to all other simulation participants in the next step).

1. Decision

2. Rationale

3. Strategy to gain staff and resident support

4. Program plans

Step 2. <u>Sharing Plans</u> (10 minutes)

As a total group of all simulation participants, share your plans by having the recorder from each group speak for that group. Give the results of your planning session: your decision; rationale; strategy to gain staff and resident support; and your program plans.

New ideas gained from the presentation of different groups:

_____

_____

_____

_____

_____

_____

_____

_____

_____

_____

_____

_____

_____

_____

_____

_____

Step 3. Debriefing (45 minutes)

Overall Questions About the Total Simulation

1. What are some of the major things you learned about psychiatric halfway houses from this simulation? What didn't you learn that you felt a need to know?

2. From what you learned about Ann McVee's job, how much fun do you think it would be to become an executive director of a halfway house? Would you rather be a staff member? A board member? Why?

3. If the simulation were true, what do you assess as the "chances" (odds) that Bridge Place would survive as a viable psychiatric halfway house?

REFERENCES

Gumrucku, P. The efficacy of a psychiatric halfway house: A three-year study of a therapeutic residence. Sociological Quarterly, 1968, 9: 374-386.

RELATED READING

Budson, R. D. The psychiatric halfway house: A handbook of theory and practice. Pittsburgh: University of Pittsburgh Press, 1977.

9

MANCOM: MANAGING A COMPREHENSIVE COMMUNITY

MENTAL HEALTH CENTER

I. INTRODUCTION

This simulation provides participants with experiences relevant to
the management of small and medium-sized comprehensive community mental
health centers. The comprehensive community mental health center is a
new and increasingly significant community agency participating in the
solution of the human problems confronting all sectors of society.
While the advancement of mental health treatment techniques has been a
primary activity of mental health professionals, there has been
considerably less attention to the problems of managing mental health
services.

The director of community mental health services must be skilled
in:

1. Managing the interrelationship among five essential
    services--inpatient, outpatient, partial hospitalization,
    emergency, and consultation/education;

2. Managing the efforts of the core mental health disciplines
    of psychiatry, psychology, social work, nursing, and
    paraprofessionals;

3. Managing the input of multiple funding sources including
    federal, state, local, voluntary, insurance, and fees;

4. Managing the coordination between services of a mental
    health center and other significant human service providers
    including public welfare, corrections, health, education,
    and law enforcement;

5. Managing the services of the mental health center with traditional mental health service providers (private practitioners and state hospitals) and with such emerging providers as halfway houses, boarding homes, nursing homes, social care homes, and foster homes.

II. GOAL AND ENABLING OBJECTIVES

Goal:

To acquaint participants with the skills necessary to manage a comprehensive community mental health center.

Enabling Objectives:

1. To gain an understanding and insight into critical community mental health issues.

2. To acquire a working knowledge of an urban community mental health center through a case study.

3. To demonstrate the ability to prioritize key administrative tasks.

4. To demonstrate the ability to derive goals and objectives for a mental health center through the involvement of senior staff (participatory management).

5. To demonstrate leadership skills in evaluating and managing client relations and staff relations.

6. To demonstrate an ability to assess critically one's own management style.

III. PROCEDURES

FRAME I - Issue Sensitizing

    Step 1. "Human Service Management Styles" (15 minutes)
    Step 2. Debriefing (5 minutes)

FRAME II - URBADEN - A Case Study of a Comprehensive Community Mental
            Health Center

    Step 1. Review Case Study (Read before beginning simulation)
    Step 2. Small Group Analysis of Urbaden Service Criteria
                (20 minutes)
    Step 3. Determining Conditions of Employment (10 minutes)
    Step 4. Group Determination of Conditions of Employment
                (20 minutes)

FRAME III - Executive Task Analysis

    Step 1. Individual Task Ranking (20 minutes)
    Step 2. Group Task Comparisons (15 minutes)
    Step 3. Task Realignment (60 minutes)
    Step 4. Debriefing (5 minutes)

FRAME IV - Goal Setting for Continuity of Care

    Step 1. Individual Development of Objectives (15 minutes)
    Step 2. Simulated Staff Meeting (45 minutes)
    Step 3. Implementing a Continuity of Care System (10 minutes)
    Step 4. Staff Meeting to Finalize Plans (15 minutes)

FRAME V - Executive Leadership Development

    Step 1. Individual Reactions to New Service Mandate (5 minutes)
    Step 2. Simulated Staff Meeting (15 minutes)
    Step 3. Staff Meeting Evaluation (25 minutes)

FRAME VI - Debriefing

    Step 1. Process and Content Reactions (30 minutes)
    Step 2. Personal Reactions (10 minutes)

FRAME I

ISSUE SENSITIZING

This initial frame is designed to sensitize participants to the
critical issues in assessing one's own management style through the use
of an inventory on "Human Service Management Styles." This instrument
will produce findings on the following dimensions: planning and goal
setting; implementation; and performance evaluation. This inventory is
based on Blake and Mouton's (1978) managerial grid concept which
describes the blend of two managerial issues.

Step 1. "Human Service Management Styles" (15 minutes)

Following this introduction are nine statements relating to
management style. Three of the statements deal with planning and
evaluation. For each statement, you are to choose the one response
which best characterizes your personal management style (your real
style, not your ideal style). When you have chosen a response that
best characterizes your personal management style, turn to the page
with the grid titled, "Human Service Management Styles." Place an "X"
in the small box which has the same number as the number of the
response you have chosen. When you have finished this exercise, you
should have nine "Xs" marked. When you have read and responded to all
the statements and placed an "X" in the appropriate box on the grid for
each response, continue with Step 2 of this frame.

HUMAN SERVICE MANAGEMENT STYLES

Planning and Goal Setting

The major goals and objectives of human service agencies are generally set by legislation, by a board of directors, or by some combination of these two. The job of the human service administrator, then, is to initiate and complete the planning necessary to achieve these larger goals and objectives. This planning process can include the identification of organizational effectiveness goals which will lead to fulfillment of the larger service goals.

ORGANIZATIONAL GOALS OFTEN DICTATE THE TYPES OF ACTIVITIES FOUND IN A HUMAN SERVICE AGENCY. ONCE THE ORGANIZATIONAL GOALS HAVE BEEN SET FOR AN AGENCY, POLICIES AND PLANS MUST BE DRAFTED WHICH WILL FACILITATE THE ACHIEVEMENT OF ORGANIZATIONAL GOALS. AS A HUMAN SERVICE ADMINISTRATOR, WHICH OF THE FOLLOWING ITEMS BEST DESCRIBES YOUR APPROACH TO THE PLANNING FUNCTION?

1. My major objective is to keep the morale of my subordinates high. Accordingly, I draft and implement policy that will satisfy this objective.

4. Since it is important to me that my subordinates and I view things in the same light, I and my subordinates work together to plan, write, and implement policy.

7. I interpret the requirements of the policy statements from legislation and/or the board of directors and develop the final plan after consulting with my subordinates.

10. My main function is to serve as a channel of communication between my superiors and my subordinates. Accordingly, I pass along the plans and objectives of my agency to my subordinates after my superiors have told me what they are.

13. In order to insure that my subordinates fully understand my expectations of them, I plan and/or interpret the objectives of my agency and then make certain that my subordinates know what I expect of them.

MANY HUMAN SERVICE ADMINISTRATORS FEEL THAT ORGANIZATIONAL EFFECTIVENESS GOALS, SUCH AS STAFF DEVELOPMENT, ARE IMPORTANT TO THE REALIZATION OF MAJOR SERVICE GOALS OF THE AGENCY. AS A HUMAN SERVICE ADMINISTRATOR, WHICH OF THE FOLLOWING BEST REFLECTS YOUR GOALS FOR STAFF DEVELOPMENT?

2. Staff development should promote the personal growth, well-being, and job satisfaction of employees within any unit of an agency.

5. Staff development has two goals, both of which are equally important: to produce a high quality of performance for the agency, and to provide an atmosphere for personal growth for the employee.

8. Once individual employees are made aware of the goals of the agency and are encouraged to participate in training programs which meet their needs, the goal of staff development has been achieved.

11. The individual employee's ambition and experience will result in personal development and so no other form of training is needed.

14. Loyal, competent, and hard-working employees are the essence of any successful agency. The goal of staff development programs should be the expansion of the knowledge and skills of such employees.

THE MONEY APPROPRIATED TO AN AGENCY SPEAKS MORE LOUDLY THAN THE LEGISLATION OR CONSTITUTION GOVERNING THAT AGENCY. HOW MONEY IS SPENT IS OFTEN MORE IMPORTANT THAN THE AMOUNT OF MONEY SPENT. WITH THESE TWO REALITIES IN MIND, WHICH OF THE FOLLOWING ITEMS BEST REFLECTS HOW YOU WOULD CARRY OUT THE RESPONSIBILITIES OF DRAFTING A BUDGET REQUEST?

3. Using last year's budget request, I would make a comparison with what was actually granted and note which areas were funded at the level of request and which areas were funded below the level of request. I would then draw up this year's budget based on that information, add my increases that might be allowed by general policies, and submit the request through normal budgeting channels.

6. I would ask all those persons whose activities are covered by my budget, and the budgeting authorities, if possible, to meet with me to discuss my agency's goals. We would then draft the budget request based on these goals.

9. I would develop a tentative budget request and have each supervisor below me identify areas of potential compromise before meeting with the budget authorities to draft the final budget request.

12. I would ask the supervisors who work below me to tell me what they need, add a small percentage for unforeseen expenses, and make this my final budget request.

15. Regardless of past budgeting policies, I would draft this year's budget request myself and then hand carry it to the budgeting authorities to explain it myself and answer any questions they might have.

Implementation

Successfully translating plans into action requires unique managerial skills. How would you, as a human service administrator, handle the implementation phase which determines whether or not your agency reaches its objectives?

YOUR AGENCY'S OBJECTIVES HAVE BEEN SET, AND THE PLANNING PROCESS TO MEET THOSE OBJECTIVES HAS BEEN COMPLETED. ALL THAT IS LEFT IS IMPLEMENTATION. WHICH OF THE FOLLOWING BEST REFLECTS HOW YOU AS A HUMAN SERVICE ADMINISTRATOR NORMALLY MANAGE IMPLEMENTATION?

16. I realize that even the most careful planning cannot anticipate all the effects plans will have on both people and production. Accordingly, I check periodically to see that my subordinates have enough leeway and are satisfied.

19. To me, implementation is just another part of planning. Therefore, my agency continues to plan as we implement.

22. I prefer to be flexible in implementation. My subordinates know that I am always available for suggestions on how to improve the implementation phase.

25. My part of implementation lies in passing on the plan for accomplishing the task and assigning responsibility. Once I have done those two things, the responsibility for task accomplishment lies with the supervisors who are below me.

28. During the implementation phase, I constantly check the progress of work and make changes as needed. My responsibility is actively to direct the work.

ONE OF THE MOST IMPORTANT PARTS OF THE IMPLEMENTATION PHASE IS
ASSIGNING RESPONSIBILITIES AND DELEGATING AUTHORITY. WHICH OF THE
FOLLOWING BEST REFLECTS HOW YOU AS A HUMAN SERVICE ADMINISTRATOR WOULD
HANDLE THE DELEGATION PROCESS?

17. Subordinates who feel qualified and who are satisfied and
    interested in certain jobs are assigned responsibility and
    authority for those jobs.

20. Personal satisfaction of employees is as important as the
    attainment of agency's objectives. Accordingly, my subordinates
    and I work together to delegate the authority necessary for each
    job.

23. I assign responsibility and authority based on my knowledge of my
    subordinates and of the job requirements. I make certain that
    everyone knows the rationale for my decisions.

26. Seniority, job descriptions, and chain of command when applicable
    determine to whom I assign responsibility and delegate authority.

29. After assessing my subordinates' unique skills and abilities, I
    assign responsibility and delegate authority on the basis of my
    assessment.

THE PROCESS USED IN HIRING PERSONNEL AND IN PROMOTING PERSONNEL ARE
SIMILAR, EVEN THOUGH THEIR FUNCTIONS ARE VASTLY DISSIMILAR. IF YOU
COULD DISREGARD OUTSIDE REQUIREMENTS (SUCH AS CIVIL SERVICE) ENTIRELY
AND HIRE AND PROMOTE PERSONNEL AS YOU WOULD LIKE, HOW WOULD YOU CARRY
OUT THIS PROCESS?

18. The potential of the position for fulfilling a person's need for
    high job satisfaction and opportunity for fulfillment would be my
    main concern.

21. Those who are concerned with the position would meet with me.
    Together we would discuss applicants' qualifications and
    interests, the requirements of the job, and then jointly select
    the person for the position.

24. I would let those involved with the positions react, evaluate
    their comments, and then make my final decision.

27. Suggestions by my superiors, or traditional organizational
    procedures, would serve as my main guideline in filling vacant
    positions.

30. I would evaluate the qualifications of people and recommend them
    for the jobs to which they seem best suited, based on my knowledge
    of the job description and the position.

Performance Evaluation

Performance evaluation is another important dimension of human service administration. Information gained from performance evaluations can be used as input for future planning, as a basis for budget requests, or to appraise the functioning of subordinates. The manner in which data are gathered, and the type of data that are gathered, can vary from evaluation to evaluation.

PRODUCTIVITY AND THE QUALITY OF WORK OF SUBORDINATES CAN BE BOTH EVALUATED AND CONTROLLED BY PERFORMANCE EVALUATIONS. ASIDE FROM AGENCY FORMS, WHICH OF THE FOLLOWING BEST REFLECTS HOW YOU AS A HUMAN SERVICE ADMINISTRATOR EVALUATE THE PERFORMANCE OF YOUR SUBORDINATES?

31. I like to ask for ways in which the conditions of a job can be improved and point out to the employee the good aspects of his/her work.

34. All my subordinates and I meet together to discuss each individual's work. I feel that this method of performance evaluation aids us in reaching both personal and organizational goals.

37. In periodic meetings with individual subordinates, I give them my personal evaluation of their performance and encourage them to ask questions so that they can begin to lay groundwork for improvement in the areas I have specified.

40. I do not personally evaluate my subordinates unless I am specifically directed to do so by my superiors.

43. I point out strengths and weaknesses and places where improvement is needed in periodic meetings with my subordinates.

RARELY DO ONE PERSON'S MISTAKES AFFECT AN ENTIRE AGENCY. BUT AN ADMINISTRATOR'S HANDLING OF ONE PERSON'S MISTAKES DOES AFFECT ORGANIZATIONAL HEALTH. WHICH OF THE FOLLOWING BEST REFLECTS HOW YOU REACT WHEN YOUR SUBORDINATES MAKE A MISTAKE?

32. The morale and self-confidence of the employee who made the mistake are very important and must not be damaged by either the mistake or any actions that result from the mistake.

35. Once a mistake is made, all of us affected by that mistake meet to discover what caused the mistake and to develop procedures to try to insure that the same type of mistake won't happen again.

38. I discipline the employee on the basis of my knowledge of the facts and then try to show him/her how he/she can learn from the mistake.

41. Unless my superiors are aware of the mistake, I don't make much of it. Mistakes are natural occurrences and are bound to happen.

44. I choose a course of disciplinary action after carefully investigating the facts surrounding the mistake.

ABILITY TO WORK WITH A PERSON DEPENDS ON HOW YOU DEAL WITH YOUR NEGATIVE FEELINGS ABOUT THAT PERSON. THE MORE NEGATIVELY YOU FEEL ABOUT SOMEONE, THE HARDER IT IS FOR YOU TO WORK SMOOTHLY WITH THAT PERSON. WHICH OF THE FOLLOWING BEST REFLECTS HOW YOU AS A HUMAN SERVICE ADMINISTRATOR NORMALLY RELATE TO SOMEONE ABOUT WHOM YOU HAVE STRONG NEGATIVE FEELINGS?

33. In an effort to become more tolerant of others, I try to work on my hostility myself without letting others know I am upset.

36. I do not want to let my negative feelings interfere with my achievement of work objectives. Accordingly, I express my negative feelings in as nonjudgmental a fashion as possible and then attempt to clear up the grievance.

39. It's important to me to know that I am not the only one bothered by this person. I ask others how they feel about this person, and if we all agree, I tell this person how we all feel.

42. In this case, avoidance is the best alternative for me. If I do have to work with the person, though, and simply can't avoid contact, I keep things "strictly business" and try to get it over with as quickly as I can.

45. I don't keep my feelings to myself; I tell the person exactly how I feel about him/her and exactly what it is that he/she is doing that irritates me.

GRID

HUMAN SERVICE MANAGEMENT STYLES

A							B	
1	2	3				4	5	6
16	17	18				19	20	21
31	32	33				34	35	36
			C					
			7	8	9			
			22	23	24			
			37	38	39			
D						E		
10	11	12				13	14	15
25	26	27				28	29	30
40	41	42				43	44	45

Step 2. Debriefing (5 minutes)

Look back to the page with the grid and count the number of "Xs" that appear in each cluster. The cluster that has the greatest number of "Xs" is your predominant management style. If two clusters have approximately the same number of "Xs," then you probably employ both styles about equally. The general significance of each of the clusters is as follows:

Cluster A - people are more important than production; "person-centered" manager

Cluster B - people and production are equally important; "ideal" manager

Cluster C - people and production are about equally balanced; "good" manager

Cluster D - neither people nor production are important; more interested in the paycheck than the job; "slide-by" manager

Cluster E - production is more important than people; "production-centered" manager.

The chart on the next page elaborates further on each type of manager's style in dealing with planning, implementation, and performance evaluation. After you complete the frames in this simulation you will have the opportunity to reevaluate your management style. Further discussion on this issue will take place in the last frame of the simulation. Use the remaining time in this step to share your impressions of this inventory with other participants before moving on to Frame II.

HUMAN SERVICE MANAGEMENT STYLES

	PLANNING (Boxes 1-15)	IMPLEMENTATION (Boxes 16-30)	PERFORMANCE EVALUATION (Boxes 31-45)
CLUSTER A	Employees' satisfaction with plans is more important to you than the quality of the plans.	Employees' job satisfaction is more important to you than the amount or quality of work they produce.	Quality of the employee is more important to you than the quality of work.
CLUSTER B	Production of the best possible plans and greatest degree of employee satisfaction with, and involvement in, those plans are equally important.	It is extremely important to you that production and morale be as high as possible.	You seek to develop the best possible qualities in your employees and, in turn, you expect them to produce the highest quality work possible.
CLUSTER C	You would like the quality of planning and employee satisfaction with those plans to be at an equal level.	Level of morale and level of production are about equally as important to you.	Both the individual and the work performed by that individual are taken into account in your evaluations.
CLUSTER D	If your supervisors hand you plans, you will pass them on to your employee.	Your main job is to direct work. You do what your supervisors tell you to do and no more.	Unless you are forced to, you don't conduct evaluations.
CLUSTER E	Plans should aim for the highest production possible.	You supervise work to make certain that production is high.	The most important aspect of any employee is how much work that employee produces.

CLUSTER A		CLUSTER B
	CLUSTER C	
CLUSTER D		CLUSTER E

FRAME II

URBADEN - A CASE STUDY OF A COMPREHENSIVE

COMMUNITY MENTAL HEALTH CENTER

Step 1. Review Case Study (adapted from Whittington, 1971)

You have just been hired as the director of the Urbaden
Comprehensive Community Mental Health Center and you are taking the
next two weeks to prepare yourself. The center is under the auspices
of the city Department of Health and Hospitals and serves a primary
catchment area of 200,000 in the northwest section of the city. Other
mental health agencies provide the full complement of the
comprehensive services in the remainder of the city and county. Four
"generic" mental health teams are decentralized into small clinic
facilities within a geographic district of the catchment area. These
teams are responsible for providing treatment and consultative services
to patients and community agencies within that district. Specialized
teams (in hospital and day hospital treatment, emergency services,
rehabilitation, and so forth) provide backup and consultative services
to the generic teams. See Figure 1 for the range of services provided.
     Basic elements of service provided are:
     1. Outpatient treatment and counseling to individuals and
         families;
     2. Brief, intensive inpatient treatment on a 24-hour basis;
     3. Partial hospitalization for patients who need structured
         hospital treatment during the day, but who are well enough
         to return home at night;
     4. Psychiatric emergency services;
     5. Consultation to other services of the hospital and to related
         mental health agencies and professionals in the community;
     6. Specialized treatment and consultative services (children,
         aged, drug addicts, etc.);
     7. Aftercare services.

Figure 1

URBADEN COMMUNITY MENTAL HEALTH CENTER

ORGANIZATION CHART

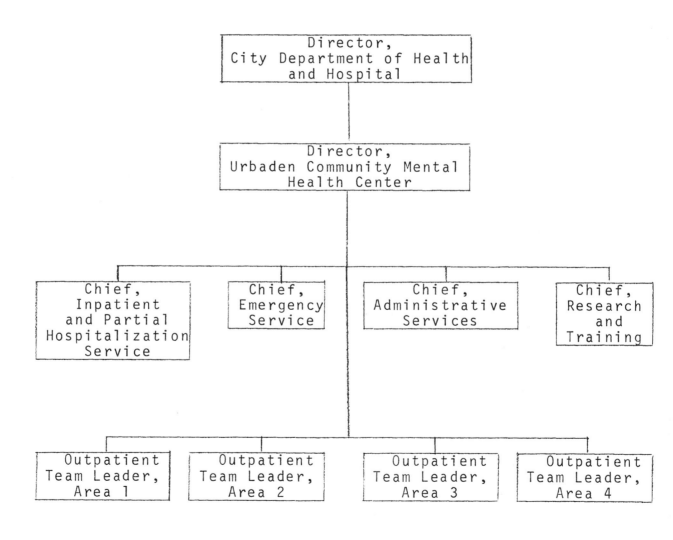

Outpatient Services

Outpatient services (including evaluation and treatment of patients and consultation to other community agencies) are provided by four teams assigned to geographic service areas of the city. Each team is directed by a psychiatrist, and composed of one or two clinical psychologists, one or two psychiatric social workers, a psychiatric nurse, a secretary-receptionist, several volunteers and/or neighborhood aides, and masters-level students in psychiatric social work and nursing.

Outpatient teams function as "psychiatric general practitioners," providing treatment to patients of all ages, with all types and degrees of illness, who reside in their service areas. The patient's first point of contact, unless he/she is seen in psychiatric consultation in another ward or clinic of the hospital, is with the outpatient team serving the area of the city where he/she lives. This team is responsible for providing, or helping the patient obtain, all services he/she needs, as long as he/she needs them.

Patients are accepted on referral from any source for outpatient evaluation and treatment of alcoholism problems. Treatment modalities include antabuse therapy, group psychotherapy, spouse group discussions, family therapy, psychoactive medications and utilization of other supportive services, such as vocational rehabilitation, Visiting Nurse Service, AA, Al-Anon, and Ala-Teens.

Hospital and Day Hospital Treatment

These two service elements are combined in a therapeutic milieu program, with a variety of large and small group, occupational, recreational, and other therapies provided for 24-hour and day patients. There are 16 beds on the hospital unit; the day program has a capacity of 24. In addition, psychiatric patients may be hospitalized in other parts of the hospital, such as the convalescent ward or the police holding unit.

Patients referred to the 24-hour or day hospital program must have a psychiatric evaluation before admission. When possible, this evaluation is conducted by the outpatient team serving the patient's area of residence, or by staff in the Emergency Room.

Average length of stay for 24-hour patients is two weeks or less. Most patients are then transferred to the day hospital program, where average length of stay is about four weeks. Patients needing 24-hour treatment for a period longer than two weeks (about one-fourth of the total caseload) are referred to the nearby state hospital.

Outpatient team members participate in small group therapy sessions, and in hospital staff conferences for treatment and discharge planning of hospitalized patients in their areas. Patients discharged from the psychiatric hospital service are automatically referred to the appropriate outpatient team for continuing treatment.

The staff of the hospital team, per se, consists of one full-time psychiatrist, two psychiatric house officers, one head nurse, seven graduate nurses, three licensed practical nurses, and seven hospital attendants. There are two social workers, one full-time and one half-time occupational therapist, one activities therapist, two secretaries, and a ward clerk. Working in partnership with the hospital team are two representatives from each of four neighborhood teams. The psychiatrist on the neighborhood teams makes rounds each morning with the hospital staff and one of his clinicians holds small group therapy with his team's group of patients two times weekly. A member of the hospital unit's nursing or social service staff serves as co-therapist for these groups.

The day care program is completely integrated with that of the 24-hour program. Most of the day care patients come five times weekly. However, frequency is individualized according to patient needs and may be no more than once weekly. Patients on day care also have the option of coming in over the weekend when they feel the need for this. Eighty percent of the day care patient group are former 24-hour care patients and about 60 percent of 24-hour care patients have a day care interval prior to discharge to the neighborhood team. Patients of all diagnostic categories are cared for in the day care program but not those who are judged to be a risk to themselves or others. A strong value of the integrated day care 24-hour care program is that the day care patients, having progressed further in their recovery, act as culture carriers for the less advanced patients.

Therapeutic programming is budgeted as follows: community meeting for total patient and staff (all), one hour per day, seven days per week; psychodrama, five hours weekly in two sessions of two hours each and one role-playing session of one hour; vocational rehabilitation, counseling, and sheltered workshop, six hours per week. The daily community meeting is felt to be most important for teaching models of problem solution and for promoting activation, resocialization, and patient-to-patient help within the community. Psychodrama is also considered by many on the staff to be the most powerful single medium for directly reaching patients psychodynamically and experientially. The two occupational therapists, the activities therapist, two members of the nursing staff, and the unit psychiatrist have had the same training in this medium and share responsibility for psychodrama sessions.

Psychotropic drugs are used very extensively. Electroconvulsive therapy is now used only very occasionally, perhaps in two or three cases per year.

Emergency Services

Many frightened, confused, and seriously mentally ill people come to the Emergency Room, at all hours of the day and night. To assure the examining intern or resident of prompt consultation in evaluating and making treatment plans for these patients, a psychiatric emergency team of four nurses and clinical psychologist are on duty in the Emergency Room and rotate shifts to provide 24-hour coverage. After completing a physical examination and preliminary evaluation, the intern may request consultation from the psychiatric emergency team if he/she thinks further investigation or treatment is needed. A team member discusses the patient and the preliminary finding with the intern and sees the patient in an evaluation interview.

Following the evaluation, the team member and intern together determine the best treatment plan and then discuss their recommendations with the patient. About one-third of the patients are referred to other private or public community agencies for continuing treatment. Others are hospitalized, referred to the appropriate outpatient psychiatric team, or carried in short-term crisis therapy by the psychiatric emergency team. Outpatient clinics of the hospital may request consultation from the psychiatric emergency team as needed.

Consultation and Education

Psychiatric consultation on Medicine, Surgery, and Ob-Gyn is provided to hospital staff on request of the primary physician, i.e., the intern or resident directly responsible for the patient's evaluation and treatment. Consultation can be either formal or informal. In informal consultation, the primary physician talks with the consulting psychiatrist about his/her patient in order to get the psychiatrist's thinking about some aspect of the case. The primary physician and consultant decide together whether the psychiatrist should see the patient. In formal consultation, the psychiatrist sees the patient and makes a thorough psychiatric evaluation.

The children's psychiatric team provides consultation and evaluation services to inpatients and outpatients of the Pediatrics Department and consults as needed with Emergency Room and outpatient psychiatric teams and with childcaring agencies in the city. Members of the children's teams are present in the Pediatric Outpatient Department during some clinic hours and are available for consultation on the ward at any time. In addition, a seminar in child psychological growth and development and a pediatric-psychiatric case conference are held each week.

In addition to consultation, outpatient teams develop and staff two advisory committees. The first is a citizen's advisory council, broadly representative of various vested-interest groups in the area, such as the ministerial alliance, the chamber of commerce, the mental health association, neighborhood groups and organizations. The purpose of this group is to help the team elicit broad community support, to keep the team informed of community sentiment and needs, and to help the team plan needed mental health programs and services. The second group is a community resources council, representing major social and

health agencies and professions in the area, formed primarily to plan
needed interagency services for multi-problem families.

Availability for public speaking in the team service area is a
way of making the team known to its constituents. Many team members
participate in the speaker's bureau and local requests for speakers are
referred to the generic team in the area.

Aftercare Services

In recent years state hospitals have embarked upon a program of
massive discharge from the overcrowded state hospital without planning
with local mental health centers. At a nearby state hospital, the
average daily census of the population had fallen from over 6,000
patients to around 2,000 patients. The majority of these chronically
and seriously ill individuals, often hospitalized for 10 to 15 years,
had been discharged to metropolitan areas. Many of them were living in
boarding homes, in which standards for care and treatment were
extremely low. Outpatient team members were also responsible for
services to these former patients.

As the new director, you are aware that all mental health centers
are periodically evaluated by state and federal officials who use the
following criteria to evaluate mental health programs. You have
learned that there are problems in each area.

A. Availability - Are services available to all persons with all
    types and degrees of illness, including evenings and weekends?

    --At Urbaden, considerable outpatient staff anxiety exists
      over the elimination of outpatient waiting lists by giving
      applicants for adult service an appointment within one or
      two days after their initial inquiry, in order to give them
      a brief appraisal interview and refer them to other
      community resources, where appropriate.

B. Accessibility - Are services accessible by public
    transportation and reachable by elevator or safe walkways?

    --At Urbaden, members of the outpatient teams have worked
      diligently to organize citizen advisory committees but
      citizens are calling for more satellite clinics in the
      neighborhoods and the staff does not know how to handle this.

C. Comprehensiveness - Is a complete range of interventive
    techniques provided, including individual counseling,
    long-term psychotherapy, family therapy, sociotherapy, group
    therapy, activity therapy, and chemotherapy?

--At Urbaden, staff have repeatedly complained about the need for more programs within the mental health center to deal with an increasing number of alcoholics referred by the police, emotionally disturbed children referred by the schools, disordered offender (criminally insane) referred by the courts, and drug addicts referred by church-sponsored rap centers.

D. Continuity of Care - Is the same outpatient clinician reponsible for initial evaluation, treatment, and follow-up of patients? Do case conferences include emergency and inpatient staff? Does the clinical record system reflect a continuity of care system?

--At Urbaden, the hospital service has refused to admit a patient upon referral from the outpatient clinic until the hospital staff "reevaluated the patient's need for hospitalization." The outpatient staff has refused, in retaliation, to allow the outpatient record to be taken from the clinic to the hospital ward, for fear that it "might get lost."

E. Quality Control - How are staff activities periodically evaluated? How often is outside consultation utilized? What type of in-service training is provided for staff?

--At Urbaden, despite the successful therapeutic community program on the inpatient service, the diffusion of responsibility for quality patient care has led to total confusion about authority with no administrative or professional accountability. Everyone's responsibility for planning case management has become no one's responsibility. This was further compounded by the recent assignment of clinical responsibility for patients to the outpatient team leader who represented the area in which the patient resided.

All these issues should be kept in mind as you proceed through the frames in this simulation.

Step 2. Small Group Analysis of Urbaden Service Criteria (20 minutes)

Divide into groups of six persons in order to discuss the case study. Particular attention should be given to the service criteria and problems noted on the previous pages. As a group, rank all five areas from "1" (most critical and therefore in need of immediate attention) to "5" (least critical), in accordance with how your group views Urbaden's problems.

Ranking	Area
_____	Availability
_____	Accessibility
_____	Comprehensiveness
_____	Continuity of Care
_____	Quality Control

Step 3. Determining Conditions of Employment (10 minutes)

Without engaging in group discussion, determine for yourself the conditions under which you would accept the position of center director if you knew what you know now about the agency. First, list the problem areas (out of the five areas previously discussed) which would make you uncomfortable in terms of your own perceptions of your competence.

1. _____

2. _____

3. _____

Now decide what guarantees you will seek (staff support, money, space, etc.) in your negotiations for the position of center director.

1. _____

   _____

2. _____

   _____

3. _____

   _____

Step 4. Group Determination of Conditions of Employment (20 minutes)

After completing your individual list, return to your previous small group and read aloud all the conditions which each participant developed and list them below. Then go through the list and by majority rule decide which conditions appear unrealistic (mark with a "U") and those that seem realistic (mark with an "R").

_____

_____

_____

_____

_____

_____

_____

This frame concludes the preliminary analysis of Urbaden and the anticipated problems confronting the selection of a new director. The objective of this frame was to apply service criteria to the problems of a mental health agency and to analyze the problems in order to set priorities in the event that you would assume the directorship of such an agency. The next frame assumes that you have been on the job several months and that you must set day-to-day priorities which overshadow the five major problem areas facing Urbaden.

FRAME III

EXECUTIVE TASK ANALYSIS

Participants will individually complete a process of prioritizing selected executive tasks which make up part of the job of a center director. Through group discussion, these tasks will be reassessed based upon alternative rankings by others. This process provides the participant with the opportunity to seek, accept, and reject the views of others and reflects a simulated consultation process whereby effective executive performance rests, in part, on the ability to solicit the views of others, especially staff members.

Step 1. Individual Task Ranking (20 minutes)

The following list of tasks was selected from a variety of tasks performed by a center director. Working individually, rank the tasks from the most important (1) to the least important (10) in the light of the problems identified in the last frame.

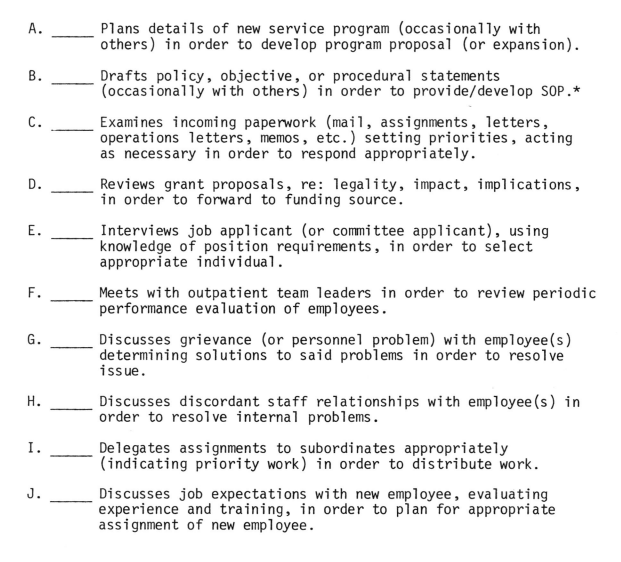

A. _____ Plans details of new service program (occasionally with others) in order to develop program proposal (or expansion).

B. _____ Drafts policy, objective, or procedural statements (occasionally with others) in order to provide/develop SOP.*

C. _____ Examines incoming paperwork (mail, assignments, letters, operations letters, memos, etc.) setting priorities, acting as necessary in order to respond appropriately.

D. _____ Reviews grant proposals, re: legality, impact, implications, in order to forward to funding source.

E. _____ Interviews job applicant (or committee applicant), using knowledge of position requirements, in order to select appropriate individual.

F. _____ Meets with outpatient team leaders in order to review periodic performance evaluation of employees.

G. _____ Discusses grievance (or personnel problem) with employee(s) determining solutions to said problems in order to resolve issue.

H. _____ Discusses discordant staff relationships with employee(s) in order to resolve internal problems.

I. _____ Delegates assignments to subordinates appropriately (indicating priority work) in order to distribute work.

J. _____ Discusses job expectations with new employee, evaluating experience and training, in order to plan for appropriate assignment of new employee.

* SOP - Standard Operating Procedures.

Step 2. Group Task Comparisons (15 minutes)

As a total group share with each other your rankings. This sharing provides for different perspectives on assessing executive functioning. Simply share your work but do not discuss.

Step 3. Task Realignment (60 minutes)

The total group will now engage in an in-basket experience in which the group members should assign themselves a number from one (1) to six (6). Then turn to the in-basket items on the next few pages according to your number (starting with the person who selected the number "1").

Each group participant should take 5 minutes to:

1. Read the in-basket item;

2. Indicate how he/she would handle the situation;

3. State the number 1 task to which you gave top priority in Step 1;

4. Field comments from group members about the fit or lack of fit between your in-basket response and your top priority task.

Other group participants should write down what is being said about the particular in-basket item which is being discussed. Move around the group until each participant has had an opportunity to respond to one in-basket item.

IN-BASKET #1

Outpatient team members are complaining that they never receive the patient records on patients transferred from the inpatient to outpatient service in sufficient time to do effective case planning. What say you?

What additional information is needed? (Everyone, except the person speaking, should fill in the blanks in writing.)

_____

_____

_____

_____

What options do you have?

_____

_____

_____

_____

What is the cost-benefit of these options?

_____

_____

_____

_____

What is your recommendation?

_____

_____

_____

_____

IN-BASKET #2

In a meeting of outpatient team leaders you learn that there is much anxiety among the teams about the no-waiting-list policy and the procedure of seeing all persons who call for help within two days. What say you?

What additional information is needed? (Everyone, except the person speaking, should fill in the blanks in writing.)

_____

_____

_____

_____

What options do you have?

_____

_____

_____

_____

What is the cost-benefit of these options?

_____

_____

_____

_____

What is your recommendation?

_____

_____

_____

_____

IN-BASKET #3

Representatives of the nurses and social workers have come to see you about the heavy-handed and part-time involvement of psychiatrists on the outpatient teams. What say you?

What additional information is needed? (Everyone, except the person speaking, should fill in the blanks in writing.)

_____

_____

_____

_____

What options do you have?

_____

_____

_____

_____

What is the cost-benefit of these options?

_____

_____

_____

_____

What is your recommendation?

_____

_____

_____

_____

IN-BASKET #4

The psychiatrists on the outpatient teams have sent you a <u>memo</u> in which they claim that consultation with other agencies and public education speeches are a waste of their valuable time. What say you?

What additional information is needed? (Everyone, except the person speaking, should fill in the blanks in writing.)

_____

_____

_____

_____

What options do you have?

_____

_____

_____

_____

What is the cost-benefit of these options?

_____

_____

_____

_____

What is your recommendation?

_____

_____

_____

_____

IN-BASKET #5

In a staff meeting with the staff of the inpatient team you learn that much confusion exists regarding the need for someone to take responsibility for treatment plans for each patient on the ward and for those in the day program. What say you?

What additional information is needed? (Everyone, except the person speaking, should fill in the blanks in writing.)

_____

_____

_____

_____

What options do you have?

_____

_____

_____

_____

What is the cost-benefit of these options?

_____

_____

_____

_____

What is your recommendation?

_____

_____

_____

_____

IN-BASKET #6

The superintendent of the nearby state hospital is on the phone complaining about the outpatient team social workers who have liaison responsibilities with the state hospital claiming that they are failing to follow-up on released state hospital patients within the 10 days specified in the original procedure agreed upon last year. What say you?

What additional information is needed? (Everyone, except the person speaking, should fill in the blanks in writing.)

_____

_____

_____

_____

What options do you have?

_____

_____

_____

_____

What is the cost-benefit of these options?

_____

_____

_____

_____

What is your recommendation?

_____

_____

_____

_____

Step 4. Debriefing (5 minutes)

Some participants should have experienced a lack of fit between their responses to in-basket items and their top-priority tasks. The in-basket items reflect the range of problems that staff bring to the director's office. The executive tasks represent the range of activities required of the director simply to maintain the administrative machinery of the center or plan for the future.

1. Do you think that the executive tasks were realistic or unrealistic?

_____

_____

_____

_____

2. Do you think that the in-basket items were realistic or unrealistic?

_____

_____

_____

_____

3. How much control should the mental health center director exercise over daily administrative demands?

_____

_____

_____

_____

FRAME IV

GOAL SETTING FOR CONTINUITY OF CARE

Since goal setting serves as a clear guide for the development of measurable objectives for all service units and support units, it affects the entire organization. In addition, clearly stated goals and objectives also serve as the basis for evaluating both the process of service delivery (treatment approaches) as well as the impact of service delivery (number of clients rehabilitated and status of functioning). Accountability for services supported by public funds continues to be a major challenge for center directors. The entire goal setting process involves: (1) stating the purpose of the mental health center; (2) deriving a set of objectives from the purpose of the agency in terms of expected output, target dates, and levels of accomplishment; (3) clustering the objectives to be met by one or more service units; (4) deriving key factors needed to measure objectives; (5) clustering of key factors to develop and operationalize indicators of center effectiveness and efficiency; (6) developing a mechanism to clarify or modify the goals of the center over time; and (7) preparing program specifications and budget information based on clearly defined goals and objectives.

Step 1. Individual Development of Objectives (15 minutes)

The new director of the center has been on the job for six months and is finally able to turn attention to the delivery issues noted at the end of the case study in Frame II (availability, accessibility, comprehensiveness, continuity of care, and quality control). The problems surrounding the continuity of care issue have surfaced repeatedly. Planning for improved continuity of care serves as the agenda for a simulated senior staff meeting involving six persons: (1) director of the center; (2) chief of inpatient services; (3) chief of outpatient services; (4) chief of emergency services; (5) budget officer; and (6) in-service training director. The director will chair the meeting, which is designed to operationalize the following policy statement:

Goal of Continuity of Care System

This system is intended to provide information to help ease the movement of patients between units and services as needed. It monitors the initiation of a transfer, the contacts made or attempted by the receiving element, and the outcome of the transfer. The information is used in making clinical decisions concerning the need to "reach out" to a patient in the community and to evaluate the adequacy of the program in providing continuous care.

Groups of six should be formed and the six roles assigned to each participant in order to role play this situation. In order to prepare for the meeting, all senior staff have been asked to develop measurable objectives for the continuity of care goal from the perspective of their position in the center. Participants should draw upon the case study in Frame II and write their objectives in the space below.

Step 2. Simulated Staff Meeting (45 minutes)

The director will chair the meeting and then begin the process of sharing statements of objectives with the ultimate objective of ending the meeting with a set of six objectives listed below that all participants can agree upon. After listing them, the group should rank order them.

_____ A. _____

_____

_____ B. _____

_____

_____ C. _____

_____

_____ D. _____

_____

_____ E. _____

_____

_____ F. _____

_____

Step 3. Implementing a Continuity of Care System (10 minutes)

In the prior steps participants developed objectives based upon a goal statement for a continuity of care system. A more complete description of a policy statement actually used in a mental health center is noted below. Review the statement before developing your plans for your participation in the next staff meeting.

The Continuity of Care System (Clarke, 1971)

I. **Goal of System.** This system is intended to provide information to help ease the movement of patients between units and services as needed. It monitors the initiation of a transfer, the contacts made or attempted by the receiving element, and the outcome of the transfer. The information is used in making clinical decisions concerning the need to "reach out" to a patient in the community, and to evaluate the adequacy of the program in providing continuous care.

II. **Characteristics of the System.** The system consists of element members who transfer a patient, the continuity of care coordinator (CCC), and the receiving element members responsible for continued care—usually the team leader, the team secretary, and a team clinician. A continuity of care form is used to record information needed to monitor the transfer process and initiate outreach attempts.

III. **Responsibility for System Functioning.** The responsibility for providing continuous care to patients resides with the director of the center. Seeing that specific patients receive the care needed is the responsibility of the receiving element, which presumably is the appropriate element for providing the care needed at that point in the patient's career. The transferring element has the responsibility of providing information to the receiving element and to the CCC. Responsibility for the overall system is delegated by the director to the CCC.

IV. **Function of the Continuity of Care Coordinator.** The CCC will monitor the transfer information concerning each patient being moved to a new service under this system. Within two days following the expiration of the suspense period for each transfer, the CCC will check for the receipt of the form; if not yet received, the CCC will telephone the receiving element and inquire into the circumstances and outreach efforts undertaken.

In the event of any failure in communication concerning the transfer of a patient, such as delay of papers, loss of papers in the mail, insufficient information to effect the transfer, etc., the CCC shall have the responsibility and authority to override established procedures and request prompt action by the receiving or sending element as needed.

V. **Publication of Transfer Success Rates and Associated Data.** Records of the outreach efforts made and outcomes of all transfers will be maintained in the CCC office. At intervals, transfer success rates for each element and each type of transfer will be calculated and distributed to team leaders and the administrator of the center.

Based on the above description of a continuity of care system, and the objectives agreed upon in Step 2, you have been asked to prepare for yet another staff meeting in which plans will be made to implement a continuity of care system. In preparing for the meeting, you should work individually in order to develop answers to the following questions:

1. Who is covered by the system (transfer) and give examples?

2. How are transfers to be initiated by the sending service unit in terms of (a) the patient, (b) forms, and (c) appropriate follow-through priority (time between origination of transfer and follow-up)?

3. How will **the receiving units** reach out to the transfer?

4. What client information regarding transfer and outreach should be recorded?

#1 _____

_____

_____

_____

#2 _____

_____

_____

_____

#3 _____

_____

_____

_____

#4 _____

_____

_____

_____

Step 4. Staff Meeting to Finalize Plans (15 minutes)

All participants should regroup to compare notes on how each person operationalized a continuity of care system for Urbaden Mental Health Center. After each person has presented his/her approach, the director should seek consensus on the following items:

1. Who is covered by the system? _____

   _____

2. How are transfers to be initiated? _____

   _____

3. How will receiving units reach out? _____

   _____

4. What patient information is needed? _____

   _____

After reaching consensus on these issues, the secretary to the director enters the conference room with an item recently received from another mental health center which outlines the details of a continuity of care system. The entire senior staff reviews a copy (see appendix) and then discusses their reactions in the light of their prior work.

APPENDIX

I. <u>Transfers Covered by the System</u>. All transfers or referrals from one service element of the center to another, except those which involve the same generic team or the same physical facility, are to be handled through the system.

EXAMPLES of Transfers Covered:

--Emergency Service to Team A Inpatient or Day Care
--Emergency Service to Team B Outpatient
--Team A Outpatient to Team B Outpatient
--Alcoholism Intake Unit to Team A Outpatient

EXAMPLES of Transfers NOT Covered:

--Team A Inpatient to Team A Outpatient
--Team A Inpatient to Team B Inpatient

Under specific arrangements, the system will cover any type of transfer occurring between the center and other psychiatric, social, or other agencies.

II. <u>Initiation of Transfer by the Sending Unit</u>. After it has been determined that further care for a patient is to be provided by another service unit in the center, the sending element should:

A. Notify the patient that he is to be seen by another unit and try to obtain his agreement to contact the new element. In the event of a transfer outside the center, obtain the patient's permission to send clinical information about him, and note this on the form.

B. Complete the Continuity of Care Form (C/C).

1. Enter the name of the sending element, the receiving element, the date of transfer, and the primary reason for transfer.

2. Enter the patient data as required.

3. Enter the clinical information required. Be concise in your description.

4. Choose an appropriate follow-through priority,
with approximate lengths of time between
origination of transfer and required follow-up
as indicated below.
URGENT - Follow-up within 2 days if possible
HIGHLY DESIRABLE - Follow-up within 5 working days
MODERATE - Follow-up within 10 working days
ELECTIVE - Follow-up within 15 working days if
   judged desirable by receiving element
OTHER - Follow-up within indicated time interval
   (indicate on form)
NOT REQUIRED - Form sent for information purposes
   only; follow-up not required

C. Send the original (white) copy of the C/C form to the
continuity of care coordinator.

D. Send the second and third copies to the receiving
element, to which the patient is being referred or
transferred.

E. Retain the fourth (blue) copy for the sending
element's files OR the sending element's patient
chart.

III. "Outreach" Procedures for Receiving Elements. Within the broad
outlines indicated below, each team will handle its continuity of
care transfers as it deems most desirable and effective. Team
leaders will prepare a written plan for handling these transfers,
to be filed with the continuity of care section and posted for
availability at the team facility. The plan will provide for
screening of mail for incoming C/C forms, relay of forms to team
member or secretary for checking against recent patient-contract
records, initial contact records, initial contact of patients by
telephone, writing to patients, requesting a home visit, and
scheduling a home visit by a team clinician as needed. The plan
will also provide for carrying out these functions if any key
person in the procedure is ill, on vacation, or otherwise not
available to handle incoming transfers.

The following should be included in each element's written plan:

A. If an "Urgent" Priority Form is received:
1. If the patient has not yet been contacted, try to
   telephone patient;
2. If there is no contact, notify the team leader;
3. Schedule a team clinician home visit immediately.

B. If a "Highly Desirable" or "Moderate" Priority Form is received:
   1. If the patient is not seen within the suspense period, try to telephone patient;
   2. If no contact is made, write the patient and again request him/her to contact the receiving element;
   3. If there still is no contact, notify the team leader, who will determine further outreach procedures, if any.

C. If an "Elective" Priority Form is received:
   1. If the patient is not seen within the suspense period, try to telephone patient;
   2. If there is no contact, notify the team leader, who will decide on further action to be taken, if any.

D. The telephone contact must be attempted first, in the interests of speed of contact and economy of effort. Home visits are expensive and limit the number of persons who can be contacted in any one day.

E. Suspense times are to be calculated from the data on the form, regardless of delays that may slow down the receipt of the form. Thus, an "Urgent" form dated May 2 and received on May 4 requires immediate action, not a delay until May 6.

IV. Recording of Transfer and Outreach Information by Receiving Element. When the final outcome has been determined, the details of the patient contact and outreach efforts are to be written on the C/C form.

   EXAMPLE: "Patient called in 5-24-78 for appointment on 5-27-78. No show. Telephone patient on 5-28-78. Patient refused to come in. Team leader discontinued outreach 5-31-78."

   One copy of the C/C form must be returned to the CCC at the center, and the other copy may be filed at the team and/or placed in the patient's chart.

FRAME V

EXECUTIVE LEADERSHIP DEVELOPMENT

No sooner has there been resolution of the continuity of care issue than word arrives of a new legislative mandate regarding another service delivery problem, quality control. The state legislation which contributes to over 40% of the Urbaden budget has recently mandated consumer involvement in the evaluation of community mental health services. Keeping the roles you played in the last frame, you have been asked to prepare for another staff meeting by completing a personal reaction form.

Step 1. Individual Reactions to New Service Mandate (5 minutes)

Before moving on to a discussion of this mandate, you should record, individually, your general reactions to the idea of having mental health service consumers evaluate the center. Consider the issues involved, recognizing that there is a wide range of possible opinions. Read all the questions on the next page and then mark your responses. Do not discuss the items with others.

Personal Reactions
(adapted from Filella & Immegart, 1971)

1. Relative to the effectiveness of the URBADEN mental health center, the request for consumer evaluation involves an issue which is:

    crucial ____; ____; ____; ____; ____ not crucial

2. Staff willingness to be evaluated by patients is the most decisive factor in involving patients in staff evaluation:

    yes ____; ____; ____; ____; ____ no

3. The value the center can realize through patient participation in evaluation is the most decisive factor in service evaluation:

    yes ____; ____; ____; ____; ____ no

4. For the center director, the evaluation of staff is:

    a major responsibility ____; ____; ____; ____; ____ not a
                                                            responsibility

5. For the staff, the evaluation of staff members is:

    a major responsibility ____; ____; ____; ____; ____ not a
                                                            responsibility

6. For the patient, the evaluation of staff is:

    a major responsibility ____; ____; ____; ____; ____ not a
                                                            responsibility

7. The overall benefits likely to accrue to the mental health center as a result of patient evaluations of staff are:

    great ____; ____; ____; ____; ____ few

8. The overall problems inherent in patient evaluations of staff are:

    great ____; ____; ____; ____; ____ few

9. Overall, as the mental health center director, I would provide leadership in order to:

    ____ a. involve patients in the evaluation of staff

    ____ b. not involve patients in the evaluation of staff

Wait until all participants have completed this page and the instructor has scanned your responses. Wait for instructions to proceed.

Step 2. Simulated Staff Meeting (15 minutes)

The next step in this frame includes a structured role-playing situation. A staff meeting has been called by the center director to discuss the role of consumers in evaluating the center's services and to reach a solution. There are only three positions to be taken on the issue: the center director (who is trying to achieve consensus); staff in favor of such evaluations (chiefs of outpatient and emergency services); and staff opposed to such evaluations (chief of inpatient, budget officer, and in-service training director). In the staff meeting, the center director should make sure that all positions have been stated and then seek a resolution to the issue.

Step 3. Staff Meeting Evaluation (25 minutes)

The primary purpose of this evaluation is to assess the role of the mental health center director. Each participant, including the one who played the center director, should complete the reaction form below (5 minutes).

Reaction Form
(adapted from Filella & Immegart, 1971)

1. In regard to patient involvement in staff evaluation, the center director's goal was:

    _____ to get a group decision to involve patients in the evaluation of the staff;

    _____ to get a group decision not to involve patients in the evaluation of the staff;

    _____ other (specify) _____

    _____.

2. At the end of the staff meeting, the decision was:

    _____ to involve patients;

    _____ not to involve patients;

    _____ other (specify) _____

    _____.

3. Respond to the following items in terms of whether your staff meeting: (1) functioned better with the center director (leadership successful); or (2) would have functioned better without the center director (leader not successful).

	(1)	or (2)
a. Directed the behavior of the group		
b. Organized the group to accomplish its task		
c. Drew out ideas of group members		
d. Focused group on task		
e. Helped group to come to its own decision		

4. How satisfied were you with the staff meeting?

    very satisfied ____; ____; ____; ____; ____ not satisfied at all
                     1   2   3   4   5

5. How constructive was the staff meeting?

    very constructive ____; ____; ____; ____; ____ not constructive
                        1   2   3   4   5   at all

6. What degree of stress or tension existed in the staff meeting?

    very high degree ____; ____; ____; ____; ____ none
                       1   2   3   4   5

    After completion, compare your observations with each other. Discuss the similarity and/or differences between your personal preferences regarding consumer involvement in evaluation noted in Step 1 and the role which you were forced to play in Step 2 (20 minutes).

FRAME VI

DEBRIEFING

Step 1. Process and Content Reactions (30 minutes)

Working backward through the simulation, discussion could focus on the following sequence of issues:

1. What is the effect of consistent or inconsistent leadership styles on group behavior?

2. What is the impact of stress on leadership styles?

3. What are critical factors in planning administrative procedures, such as those for continuity of care?

4. Why is goal setting a difficult process?

5. What is the relationship between the tasks of the executive and the goals of a mental health center?

6. How might the organizational problems of an urban mental health center differ from a rural center?

Step 2. Personal Reactions (10 minutes)

1. Turn to the next page and copy the diagram on a blank sheet of paper and write your name at the top. Now pass your paper around the group so that each participant can place an "x" in the box which best reflects his/her view of your management style throughout this simulation.

2. How do your self-perceptions from Frame I compare with those observations of other participants regarding your concern for people and for production?

_____
Name

HUMAN SERVICE MANAGEMENT STYLE

A Person- Centered		B Ideal
	C Good	
D Slide- By		E Production- Centered

Concern for People ↑

⟶ Concern for Production ⟶

REFERENCES

Blake, R. R., & Mouton, J. S. The new managerial grid. Houston, Tex.:
Gulf Publishing Company, 1978.

Clarke, J. Continuity of care system. In Whittington, H. G. (Ed.),
Development of an urban mental health center. Springfield, Ill.:
Charles C Thomas, 1971, pp. 191-199.

Filella, J., & Immegart, G. C. Exercise VI: Leadership. In
ED/AD/EX. Scottsville, N. Y.: Transnational Programs Corp.,
1971.

Whittington, H. G. (Ed.). Development of an urban mental health
center. Springfield, Ill.: Charles C Thomas, 1971, pp. 22-24,
41-52, 56-72, 101-109.

RELATED READINGS

Feldman, S. (Ed.). The administration of mental health services.
Springfield, Ill.: Charles C Thomas, 1973.

Schatz, H. A. A casebook in social work administration. New York:
Council on Social Work Education, 1970.

10

THRONATEESKA: MANAGING A STATE MENTAL HOSPITAL

John Whiddon

I. INTRODUCTION

Large institutions are, within themselves, communities. Those
large institutions which are also residential in nature are very much
like cities. They require laws, maintenance, physical care, planning,
coordination, and all the other functions which keep a metropolis
running. Thus, the administrator of a large state mental institution
operates in very much the same fashion as does a city manager.

Many skills are needed to be an effective city manager, as well as
a broad knowledge base. One of the key ingredients for a successful
administrator is flexibility--the ability to switch gears often
throughout the day, to change as the situations and demands change.

The purpose of this simulation is to teach participants some of
the content and the processes involved in managing an institutional
community. Participants will experience a day in the life of the busy
superintendent of Thronateeska State Hospital, a large state mental
hospital. They will learn the importance of flexibility and the
ability to switch from one problem to another during the work day of an
institutional mental health administrator.

II. GOAL AND ENABLING OBJECTIVES

Goal:

To acquaint participants with the knowledge and skills
which are necessary for managing an institutional
community successfully.

Enabling Objectives: Participants will be able to:

1. Develop a structure for decision making;
2. Set priorities;
3. Mediate peer conflict;
4. Delegate work to subordinates;
5. Deal with subordinates' errors and settle resulting
    internal disturbances.

III. PROCEDURES

INTRODUCTION TO THE THRONATEESKA COMMUNITY

FRAME I - Developing a Structure for Decision Making

    Step 1. Choosing Roles and Reviewing Existing Policy (15 minutes)
    Step 2. Staff Meeting (30 minutes)
    Step 3. Debriefing (20 minutes)

FRAME II - Setting Priorities

    Step 1. Individual Prioritizing (20 minutes)
    Step 2. Group Prioritizing (20 minutes)
    Step 3. Debriefing (20 minutes)

FRAME III - Mediating Peer Conflict

    Step 1. Sorting Out the Issues (20 minutes)
    Step 2. Taking Action (20 minutes)
    Step 3. Debriefing (20 minutes)

FRAME IV - Delegating Work to Subordinates

    Step 1. Collective Executive (20 minutes)
    Step 2. Classifying Responses (15 minutes)
    Step 3. Comparing Responses (20 minutes)
    Step 4. Debriefing (20 minutes)

FRAME V - Staff Problem Solving

    Step 1. Assigning Roles and Conducting the Meeting (30 minutes)
    Step 2. Debriefing (20 minutes)

INTRODUCTION TO THE THRONATEESKA COMMUNITY

Effective management requires knowledge of many aspects of an institution. A good superintendent should be familiar with his/her job description, the persons holding key positions in the institution, the historical perspective of the institution, and the organizational structure (both formal and informal) of the institution.

Thronateeska is one of the public mental hospitals in the state. The job description for superintendent is standard for each of the institutions and, like most job descriptions for upper level management, it is somewhat vague. The superintendent's job is one which is highly professional and involves considerable responsibility in directing the operations of a state mental hospital. The superintendent is responsible for supervising the operations of all hospital personnel; formulating, recommending, and implementing new policies and procedures, conducting and supervising the institution's program as directed, and advising administrative personnel regarding the policies and procedures to be followed. Superintendents of institutions such as Thronateeska are directly responsible to the governor's designee for mental health and human service administration.

The former superintendent administered Thronateeska during the last 22 years of his 45 years of employment with the state. He was a tall, stately man with silver-white hair who always spoke slowly and softly. Underneath his leisurely ways and Southern manners lay a mind like a steel trap. He himself attended every session of the legislature, speaking for Thronateeska rather than allowing the governor's representative to do it for him. The new superintendent was recently chosen and was due to spend the next two weeks at Thronateeska in order to learn more about the hospital, its staff, and the surrounding area. Thronateeska is located in a small town, fairly isolated (70 miles) from the nearest city. The major source of employment for the town's 5,200 residents is the hospital. Most of the residents were born in the town, as were their parents. The rest of the town's population is foreign-born, moving to the town to assume professional positions at the hospital.

Prior to becoming a state hospital, Thronateeska had been a
Spanish arsenal and later a state penitentiary. In 1876 it was
converted into a state hospital, bearing the name Thronateeska State
Hospital for Indigent Lunatics. Prior to 1876, the mentally ill were
kept in the neighboring state and when the hospital was opened they
were brought down the nearby river by boat.

Since that time the size of the hospital and the number of
patients has increased. In 1944, when Thronateeska was still the only
one of its kind in the state, reports showed that the state owned
10,278 acres of land for its operation. There were 288 buildings,
5,203 patients, and 793 employees. Presently there are 14,278 acres of
land for its operation, 305 buildings, 5,023 patients, and 2,503
employees.

Thronateeska, in the tradition of most of the early mental health
institutions, is geographically isolated from major population centers
in the state. It has always been difficult to recruit and maintain a
highly trained professional staff. This has resulted in a strong
informal organizational structure composed of longtime local employees.

This kind of informal organization is the way things are
accomplished at Thronateeska and for the most part it ignores the
legitimate power structure. Nepotism is a fact of life at
Thronateeska. Without employing people that were related to each other
there would be few people employed at the hospital.

The hospital operates entirely on the medical model and the key
actors in the system are the nurses with longevity and seniority. The
major organizational charts appear on the following pages.

By law Thronateeska is supposed to provide treatment and care for
the psychotic. Over the years, however, the hospital has become a
final depository for anyone that society has no adequate programs or
facilities for. The client population at Thronateeska includes people
in the following categories: psychotic; geriatric; organic brain
syndromes; sociopathic personalities; blind; diabetic; retarded; and
drug addicted.

The hospital functions and operates in two major ways: treatment and maintenance. Treatment includes chemotherapy, group counseling, occupational therapy, music therapy, and recreation. Maintenance includes all the support and ancillary services needed to feed, clothe, and house patients at the hospital.

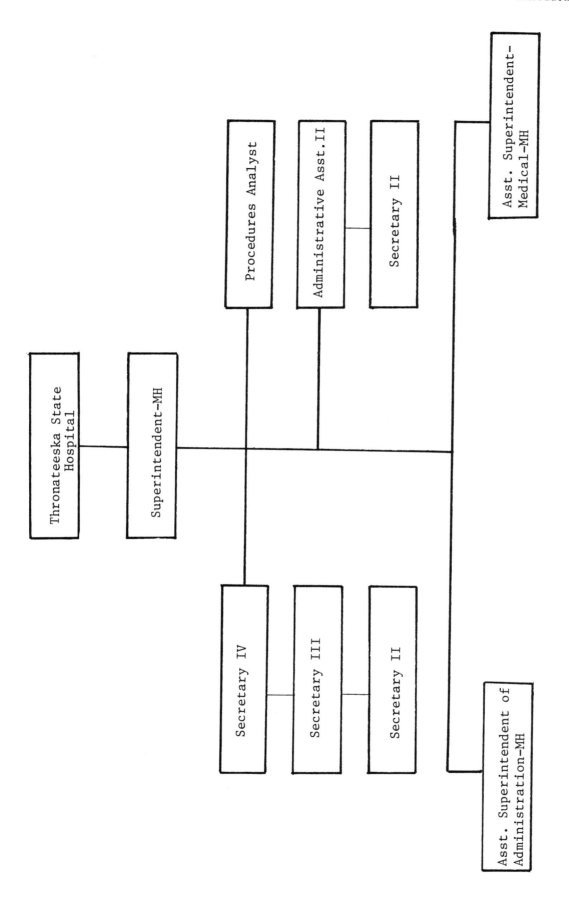

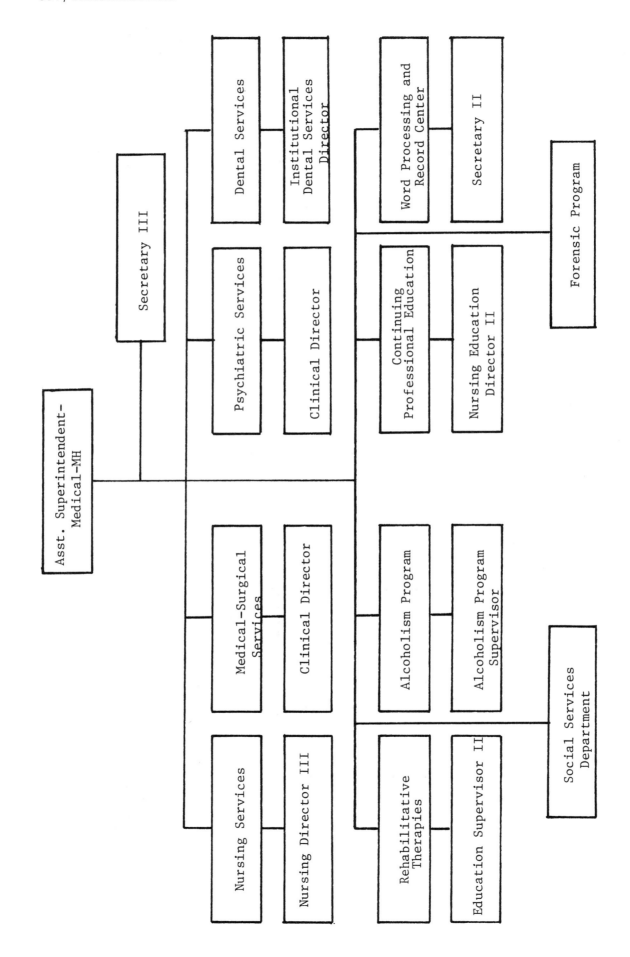

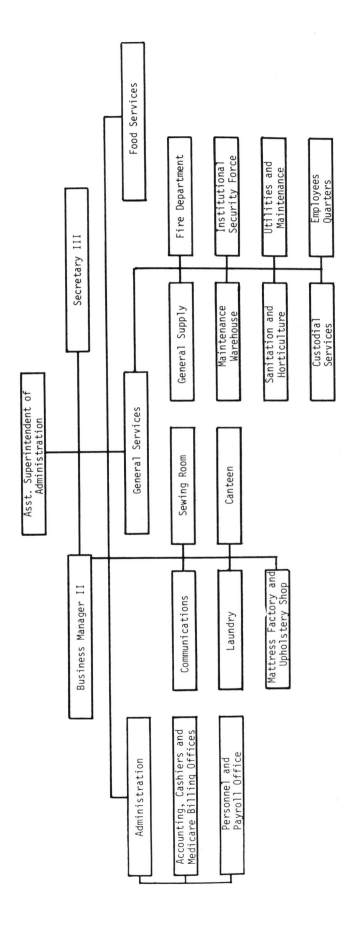

FRAME I

DEVELOPING A STRUCTURE FOR DECISION MAKING

Dr. Tom Blau is the new superintendent of Thronateeska. Dr. Blau arrived on July 8, five days after the death of the previous superintendent. He is unfamiliar with the current methods of operation of the hospital, having spoken with the governor's mental health representative during his interviews. He does not know any of the staff and has had to call them into his office to introduce himself and to meet them. The staff he has met so far have been polite but seemingly suspicious or hostile. He found his first day on the job to be a bit lonely, and he is wondering if he will ever make any friends in this small, tightly-knit town. He realizes that the memory of the former superintendent is still very, very strong, and that the staff seems to be intent upon keeping the hospital operating exactly as it was done under the former superintendent.

In addition to the troubles inherent in being new, Dr. Blau is faced with a minor crisis that is scheduled to occur during the morning of his second day on the job. Just before he left for Thronateeska, Dr. Blau received a call from the governor's mental health representative. Recent scandals over escaped forensic patients have created an uproar, and the legislature has recently taken action which requires a review of ground privileges for forensic patients. On his first day at Thronateeska, Dr. Blau's administrative assistant informs him that the biweekly senior staff meeting is scheduled for the next day. Dr. Blau plans to deal with the agenda item dealing with forensic patients.

In this frame, you will be dividing yourselves into groups of seven to role-play the staff meeting mentioned above, in which the prime goal is to assign someone to respond to the legislative action by reviewing the hospital's policy concerning ground privileges for forensic patients. Dr. Blau and his staff are to work together to develop a structure for making a decision about the grounds privileges issues. A few decision criteria should be kept in mind by participants as they work through the staff meeting:

1. Who can do the job best?

2. What would be the ideal system?

3. What alternatives exist for changing or modifying the system?

4. Does the proposed system insure always, sometimes, or never that the situations will be resolved appropriately?

Step 1. Choosing Roles and Reviewing Existing Policy (15 minutes)

Each of you should choose one of the following roles:

Dr. Tom Blau, Superintendent

Mary Hadi, Assistant Superintendent, Administration

Dr. Jack O'Sullivan, Assistant Superintendent, Medical

Dr. Heather McVoy, Director of the Forensic Program

Dr. Robert Lagos, Clinical Director of Psychiatric Services

Mark Hinson, Director of the Social Services Department

Max Lawrence, Business Manager

When each of you has selected his/her role, turn to the following two pages and read the material on the existing policy at Thronateeska.

When each of you has finished reading the material, proceed to the next step.

Policy 123

Forensic patients being considered for grounds privileges must go through a process that entails two steps. First of all, the court must decide whether or not to permit ground privileges. If the court allows it, a staff evaluation (outline noted below) must be completed with primary attention given to the character and performance of the patient. The type of crime and public reaction are secondary. Staff members involved in granting grounds privileges include:

--Superintendent of Thronateeska;
--Assistant Superintendent, Medical;
--Clinical Director, Psychiatric Services;
--Head of Forensic Program.

Staff deliberations shall be based upon, but not limited to, a report prepared by the social worker who has been working with the individual patient.

Conditions for Determination by the Staff of Thronateeska of the Granting of Grounds Privileges to Forensic Patients

I. Security Concerns
   A. Degree of Dangerousness
      1. History of aggressive behavior
      2. Nature of crime
      3. Past criminal record, with assaultiveness to others being an important factor
      4. Behavior on ward
      5. Relative cooperativeness

   B. Type of Security Risk
      1. To other patients/staff
      2. To self
      3. To facility image
      4. To society at large

   C. Degree of Security Risk
      1. History of previous escapes and attempted escapes
      2. Conditions surrounding escapes

II. Motivation and Response to Treatment
  A. Involvement in Program Ward Activities
  B. A Specific Therapeutic Aim Must be Stated in Order to Justify the Granting of Additional Freedom of Movement
  C. Client Articulation
III. Nature of Crime Resulting in Institutionalization
  A. Notoriety of Crime
  B. Public Sentiment

Step 2. Staff Meeting (30 minutes)

Each of you should turn to the appropriate page which contains your role description. Read only your role description. When each participant has read his/her role description, Dr. Blau should open the meeting by identifying himself and stating briefly what his perspective is on the issue. Each member of the staff should then briefly identify him/herself and give his/her perspective. When all staff members have spoken, Dr. Blau should lead the discussion toward a review of the policy on ground privileges for forensic patients and a resolution of the policy issue.

When your group has completed this role play, proceed to the next step.

Role Description for <u>Dr. Tom Blau</u>, Superintendent

This is your second day as superintendent of Thronateeska. You are familiar with the broad outlines of the issue, but you feel that some persons on your staff should have more expertise in this area than you do. Your wish is not to dominate the discussion, but rather to guide it so that you can get a good idea of what each individual is like. You have three objectives for this meeting:

1. To air feelings and views;
2. To delegate the drafting of a revised statement to the most appropriate senior staff member;
3. To set a time limit on staff completion.

Role Description for <u>Mary Hadi</u>, Assistant Superintendent
  of Administration

You have worked in administration for a number of years and know all the "ins and outs." You have been at Thronateeska for four years, and you have found it hard to be accepted as a professional because you were the first woman employed in upper level management. You are eager to support Dr. Blau, as you feel that he will bring some new ideas and approaches to the hospital. You also hope that he will, in turn, provide you with more support than the previous superintendent. Your view of ground privileges for forensic patients is that Thronateeska should proceed somewhat slowly, checking with the other state hospitals to see what their stands on this issue are. You realize that handling this potentially explosive issue is crucial to the success of Dr. Blau as superintendent of this hospital. Although you know that any type of decision made two days after Dr. Blau's arrival is not a fair indication of his ability, you know that others will be judging him on just this one decision.

Role Description for <u>Dr. Jack O'Sullivan</u>, Assistant
  Superintendent, Medical

     You have been at Thronateeska for 15 years in your present
position. You and the former superintendent were close friends, and he
had groomed you to take over his position upon his retirement. You
were, needless to say, disappointed when his job was not offered to
you. You agreed with just about everything that the former
superintendent developed and you are intent upon continuing his
policies in the future. In relation to grounds privileges for forensic
patients, what is most important to you is that the legislature not be
angered or upset by any action taken by Thronateeska. The former
superintendent worked hard to gain special relationships with many of
the older legislators, and you do not want to see these relationships
disturbed. Accordingly, you want to be as conservative as possible in
your approach on this issue.

Role Description for <u>Dr. Heather McVoy</u>, Director of the
  Forensic Program

     You have been employed at Thronateeska for two years, ever since
you completed your graduate training. You were pleased to get this
job, as it is unusual for any recent graduate (particularly a woman) to
be offered such a degree of responsibility. You have not been able to
implement many of the ideas you developed in school concerning the
treatment of forensic patients and you are hoping that you will be able
to do so under Dr. Blau. On the issue of grounds privileges for
forensic patients, you would like the policy to be much more liberal
than it is now. You would also like grounds privileges to be more of a
day-to-day matter, so that it could be incorporated into a behavior
modification program you would like to try. This means that counselors
and social workers in your program would have a greater determination
in grounds privileges than would senior staff.

Role Description for <u>Dr. Robert Lagos</u>, Clinical Director
  of Psychiatric Services

You have been employed at Thronateeska for eight years. You were
promoted to your present position two years ago. Your actual contact
with the patients has decreased almost to zero. Most of your time is
devoted to administrative work (assignment of budgetary matters, etc.).
You would like to have more harmony among the staff members, as there
is a split between the older, more conservative members of your staff
and the younger, more liberal members. The resolution of the issue is
not as important to you as having the staff members be satisfied with
the decision. You would like to get input from those who work with the
forensic patients and those who work with the legislature, and then
balance the two inputs to derive a solution that is best for both.

Role Description for <u>Mark Hinson</u>, Director of the Social
  Services Department

You hope that, under Dr. Blau's administration, your department
can become more influential in treatment of patients. You feel that
the doctors often have too much authority and you would like to see
models other than the medical model used in this hospital. You have
become particularly tired of the "This is how we've always done it"
viewpoint. In relation to the issue of grounds privileges for forensic
patients, you think that you should have a fairly large hand with
formulating the new policy.

Role Description for <u>Max Lawrence</u>, Business Manager

You have been employed at Thronateeska for the last 18 years, and you are looking forward to your retirement. You liked your relationship with the former superintendent and you hope that you won't have to make too many changes for Dr. Blau. Your job and your life are fairly comfortable, and you don't want to see them disrupted. You don't have any particular bias in relation to the issue of grounds privileges for forensic patients, but you realize the importance of not alienating the legislature. If the legislature is alienated, the funding for the hospital will undoubtedly suffer. You would not like to see that happen.

<u>Step 3. Debriefing</u> (20 minutes)

Working within your entire group, answer the following questions:

1. What are some guidelines for developing a structure for decision making? Is the person closest to the problem or issue the best person to involve in the solution?

2. What role should the chief administrator play in developing a structure for decision making? Should he make his own views crystal clear or seek to bring out all the views reflected around the table?

3. What role does self-interest have in the actions of those other than the chief administrator? Can you satisfy the self-interest of staff at the same time as you seek the best option for the patients?

FRAME II

SETTING PRIORITIES

You have just returned from the staff meeting on the forensic policy and you notice that your administrative assistant, Terri, has filled your in-basket with several sheets of paper. In this frame, you will set priorities that will aid you in deciding what priority you will give to each of these matters.

Step 1. Individual Prioritizing (20 minutes)

Working by yourself, read the in-basket items found on the following pages. After reading all the items, divide them into "routine" matters and "nonroutine" matters. Once each item has been placed in either one of the categories, rank order the items within each category. Assign "1" to the item you feel is most important, "2" to the second most important item, and so on. Use the following space to divide the items and rank-order them.

When everyone has finished this step, proceed to the next step.

ROUTINE		NONROUTINE	
Rank	In-basket #	Rank	In-basket #

In-Basket #1

STATE DEPARTMENT OF HEALTH
AND REHABILITATION
Division of Mental Health
Health and Welfare Building
State Capital

July 9, 1978

Dr. Tom Blau, Superintendent
Thronateeska State Hospital

Dear Superintendent:

I hope your brief tenure at Thronateeska State
Hospital has been personally and professionally
meaningful. By this time you have probably had time to
analyze the administrative structure and program created
by the former superintendent.

Prior to your arrival, I had an opportunity to
conduct a site visit. Changes need to be made at
Thronateeska if we are to provide effective services for
the residents. These changes must be in line with
contemporary trends in mental health philosophy and
programming.

I hope to be by your office this Friday following a
presentation I'm scheduled to make to the Mental Health
Association. I would like to discuss the following issues
with you:

1. Plans for any administrative restructuring
of Thronateeska State Hospital

2. The treatment philosophy of Thronateeska
State Hospital in terms of the "principle
of normalization"

3. Possible alternatives to institutionalization
in the Thronateeska County area

Hopefully we will discuss the above topics this
Friday. If not, I'll arrange to meet with you next week.

Sincerely,

David Webster

David A. Webster, Director
Division of Mental Health

DAW:io

In-Basket #2

MEMORANDUM

TO: Max Lawrence, Director of
        Management Services

FROM: Diane Heller, Accountant *DH*

RE: ESEA Title I Account #3931

DATE: July 1, 1978

    In reviewing ESEA Title I account #3931, I have
found $230,000 of unencumbered funds. This money is a
grant award designated by law to be spent on instructional
equipment and materials to be used specifically by the
Education and Training Program. The funds must be spent
for their designated purpose within the next 30 days or
returned to the funding agency.

DH:io
cc: Dr. Tom Blau, Superintendent
     Jack Manson, Accountant
     Leroy McIntosh, Director of
        Education and Training

In-Basket #3

MEMORANDUM

TO: Dr. Blau, Superintendent

FROM: John Wells, President
        Employees' Local 905 AFL-CIO

RE: Suspension of a union member

    One of our union members, Alomee Zentivloich, has
been suspended from work for three days by James Thomas,
the Personnel Director. The charges are stealing food
from kitchen stores. Since this is a union matter, I
want you to forward to me all the details of the case, a
copy of Mr. Zentivloich's personnel folder, and the
formal complaints that have been filed.

JW:io

In-Basket #4

MEMORANDUM

TO: Dr. Tom Blau, Superintendent

FROM: L. McIntosh, Director of Training *LMI*
        and Education

RE: Staff Meetings

DATE: July 9, 1978

    Please excuse the frankness of this memo, but I have
something that I have to get off my chest. As director
of the Education program here at the institution, my
influence at the regular staff meetings has been less
than significant. It should be obvious to you that these
"staff" meetings continue to be medical staff meetings
with the remainder of the staff sitting in as observers.

    I would like you to do what I have done. Keep track
of the conversations at these meetings. Observe who makes
the decisions and to whom others address themselves when
asking for a decision.

    I still believe that education is the primary and not
secondary function of this institution. When will we
finally drop the medical model?

LMI:ia

In-Basket #5

2725 Wood Lawn Avenue
Oak Lawn   90371

July 3, 1978

Dr. Tom Blau, Superintendent
Thronateeska State Hospital
Rio Tatuo, Florida

Dear Dr. Blau:

　　Recently we visited our son, Jerry. Jerry is a
patient in W-2. He has been doing very well since being
admitted to Thronateeska. We visit him very frequently.
We are very distressed, however, because of the declining
conditions of one of the other residents in W-2. The
resident who occupies the bed next to our Jerry, according
to the attendant, never gets any visitors. This young man
seems very, very depressed and frequently cries for his
parents. My husband and I just feel so sorry for him. It
appears that he has not been eating, and the attendant
tells us that he acts out frequently. We are very worried
about him, and if there is anything we can do personally,
we would like to. We are hoping that you can look into
this situation.

　　Are we allowed to visit with him just like we visit
with our Jerry? We are willing to do this if it will help
the man. Please advise us.

Sincerely,

Mrs. James Fincher

In-Basket #6

July 9, 1978

Chief Stigger from the City Police Department came to the office yesterday and indicated that it was urgent that he set up a meeting with you as soon as possible.

Terri

Administrative Assistant

In-Basket #7

Honorable Jim Knight
Judge, 5th Circuit Ct.
Banana County, Florida

Dr. Tom Blau, Superintendent
Thronateeska State Hospital

Dear Dr. Blau:

    I realize that you are new at Thronateeska but I feel
that I must make a point and maybe now is the most
appropriate time. I am tired of playing ping pong with
your patients. It is not in the best interest of the
court's time or the hospital's time to send patients under
the jurisdiction of the court back to the court when they
are not ready to be sent back. That is why I sent them to
your hospital to begin with. I feel that if you would
spend half as much time trying to treat them as you do
trying to get rid of them that you would probably achieve
outstanding results.

    One thing for sure. The next time you send me a
mentally disordered sex offender that has been at the
hospital for less than a year I'll subpoena every staff
member at your hospital that has ever been in contact with
the patient to appear and testify at the hearing.

                          Yours truly,

                          Jim Knight

                          Jim Knight

JK:ia

In-Basket #8

MEMORANDUM

TO: Tom Blau, Superintendent

FROM: Robert Lagos, Clinical Director **R. Lagos**

RE: Reorganization

DATE: July 9, 1978

We need to begin thinking about the possibility of reorganizing our medical and psychiatric services in light of anticipated legislative action. I really think it would be a good idea to make this a top priority item in order that we can get a good jump on any new program requirements.

I have spoken to Dr. O'Sullivan about this and he endorses my opinion.

RL:cg
cc: Dr. O'Sullivan

In-Basket #9, #10, #11 . . . . .

Dr. on Call Report (Dr. Burns) 8 a.m. - 5 p.m. July 7, 1978. (If necessary, treat each item in this report as a separate in-basket item.)

Incident Report

8:45   Patient (pt.) Martha Jo Henry admitted from Escambia County (routine admission).

9:20   Firecrackers exploded in east side of G. Building. No injuries, no damages. Small boys seen running from area.

9:50   Pt. Eda Bromfield delivered baby boy John Bromfield, 8½ lbs. Baby and mother fine. Family notified, DFS notified.

10:30   Disturbance in Diet Kitchen, Pt. John Morgan acting out. Pt. was restrained and given appropriate PRN order.

11:04   Fire alarm accidentally went off in Plumbing and Electrical supply. Fire Department and Security investigating cause.

11:25   Pt. Adam Higgins, age 74, expired on medical surgical. Apparent natural causes, family notified.

11:45   Pts. Eddie Fields, Tom McRay escaped taking Aide Tom Adkins as hostage. Adkins was released as two left the building. Security Force and local authorities contacted.

12:10   Pt. Tom McRay returned and readmitted to hospital.

12:35   Pt. Tom McRay taken to medical surgical for stitches and broken wrist. Pt. fell in bathroom.

1:50   Toilet flooded in W-2 Unit. Plumber called.

3:00   Pt. Betty Phillips returned from Liberty County from trial visit. Parents brought her. Pt. actively hallucinating. Ran from building, was apprehended and admitted.

(continued on next page)

3:10   Nurse treated in emergency medical surgical for deep cut and lacerations obtained from admitting Pt. Phillips.

3:55   Pt. Tom Moorse expired on W-2 from apparent reaction to sodium amythal administered during massive seizure. Autopsy ordered.

4:32   Security reported parked car on hospital grounds behind maintenance shed. Owner was not located. Local authorities called to investigate.

5:00   Relieved by Dr. Perry.

Step 2. Group Prioritizing (20 minutes)

Rejoin the group with which you worked in Frame I. Let each
member quickly read his/her rank ordering of routine and nonroutine
items. Then, as a group, decide which items are routine and
nonroutine, and then rank order the items within each of the
categories. It is not necessary to gain a unanimous decision on each
and every item. What is important is to hear each member's reason for
placing the item as he/she did. Note the group decision below.

When your group has finished this step, proceed to the next step.

ROUTINE   NONROUTINE

Rank	In-basket #	Rank	In-basket #

Step 3. Debriefing (20 minutes)

Staying within your group, answer the following questions:

1. Did your individual classifications and rankings differ markedly from the group's classifications and rankings? If so, what do you think this means in terms of your own priorities?

2. Did the group use any specific criteria in classifying and/or ranking the items? If so, what were they?

3. Now that all the items are classified and ranked, what is next? That is, as Superintendent Blau, would you deal with all the nonroutine items before taking up any of the routine items? Or would you alternate between routine and nonroutine items? Why?

FRAME III

MEDIATING PEER CONFLICT

You have just finished prioritizing all the items in your
in-basket. Looking at your watch, you see that most of your morning
has gone, and you are hoping to spend the time before lunch reviewing
some of the material that was left in the files of the former
superintendent. Terri, your executive assistant, taps on your door
and tells you that Dr. McVoy, who is head of the forensic program, and
Dr. Lagos, the clinical director of psychiatric services, are outside
and would like to see you. You ask if it's urgent and she replies that
they both look kind of agitated and upset. You say you will see them.

Dr. McVoy enters the room first, shakes your hand, and takes the
chair closest to your desk. As soon as Dr. Lagos has finished shaking
your hand, Dr. McVoy begins to speak: "Dr. Blau, as you probably know,
the job specifications for the position of psychiatric aide are being
rewritten. I feel it is most important that the aspects of a
therapeutic community be included in the description--that the aides
have a say in patient treatment, ward routine, and the like. They are
capable of and should do more than serve as servants of the nurses. If
this hospital is to become progressive, I must retain the right to use
my staff as I see fit. And this means that my suggested corrections
must be included in the job specifications for psychiatric aide. If
you will give me a few minutes of your time, I will be glad to explain
my reasoning, and I'm sure you'll agree."

During her speech, you notice that Dr. Lagos has been squirming
around in his chair. You say, "Thank you, Dr. McVoy. I'd like to hear
from Dr. Lagos also, so that I may gain a clear picture of exactly what
is happening here. I'd appreciate it if you two could give me more of
the background behind this situation."

Dr. Lagos starts to speak with a slight Spanish accent, "Dr. Blau,
as you know, psychiatric aides have been an integral part of the
treatment process at Thronateeska. It's just that I'm not too sure we
should rush into changing things. This job description will apply to
my wards as well as the forensic unit, and I think it ought to be as

general as possible, to cover all possibilities. I think it would be just as wrong to force someone else into following Dr. McVoy's program as it would be to force Dr. McVoy to follow someone else's program. I'm sure you agree that we have room for both uniformity and new ways of doing things here at Thronateeska, based on your practices of what we know works well. I just can't see change for the sake of changing."

After talking with each of them for a few minutes and asking them direct questions, you get a clearer idea of what they are arguing about and the background: a new job description for the position of psychiatric aide must be drafted, as a part of the total civil service revision of job specifications. Thronateeska has been asked to submit a draft of a proposed revision by September 1. The personnel director worked up the draft and then sent it to Drs. Lagos and McVoy for their suggested changes, if any. Apparently psychiatric aides are used very differently by Dr. Lagos and Dr. McVoy. Dr. Lagos uses them in a more traditional manner, to escort patients to therapy, to restrain unruly patients, and the like. Dr. McVoy involves them in staff meetings, where they are encouraged to give their opinions on all the matters being discussed by the staff, rather than simply implementing the decisions of others.

Dr. McVoy changed the job description to include the functions performed by her psychiatric aides and returned the draft to the personnel director. Dr. Lagos did not change his draft at all and returned it to the personnel director. The personnel director sent both drafts to Dr. Lagos, with a memo asking him to settle the differences and return the final product to him. The memo was sent by carbon copy to Dr. O'Sullivan, assistant superintendent medical, and to Dr. McVoy.

After this morning's staff meeting on grounds privileges for forensic patients, Dr. Lagos brought up the matter to Dr. McVoy. They have been arguing about it ever since. They first tried to get Dr. O'Sullivan, but he had left his office for an early lunch. They then came to your office.

<u>Step 1. Sorting Out the Issues</u> (20 minutes)

Divide into groups of six persons each. Within each of these groups, choose one of the following roles (be sure that the first three roles are taken before choosing one of the last three roles):

--Dr. Blau;

--Dr. McVoy;

--Dr. Lagos;

--Observer #1;

--Observer #2;

--Observer #3.

To prepare yourself, refer to the organizational charts in the Introduction. Also turn to one of the following pages which correspond to the role you have chosen. Work alone by reading and answering each of the questions for your role. Do not look at any of the other roles.

When all members of your group have finished this step, proceed to the next step.

DR. BLAU

1. What are the main issue(s) for Dr. McVoy?

   _____

   _____

2. What are the main issue(s) for Dr. Lagos?

   _____

   _____

3. Exactly what is the problem, as you see it?

   _____

   _____

4. Exactly what are you being asked to do?

   _____

5. How soon does this problem need to be solved?

   _____

6. Are you the one to solve it? _____

   If not, who is?_____

7. The solution to this problem should be _____

   _____

   _____

DR. McVOY

1. What are the main issue(s) for you?

    _____

    _____

2. What are the main gripe(s) about Dr. Lagos?

    _____

    _____

3. Exactly what is the problem, as you see it?

    _____

    _____

4. Exactly what are you asking Dr. Blau to do?

    _____

    _____

5. How soon does this problem need to be solved?

    _____

    _____

6. The solution to this problem should be _____

    _____

    _____

DR. LAGOS

1. What are the main issue(s) for you?

   _____

   _____

2. What are the main gripe(s) about Dr. McVoy?

   _____

   _____

3. What is the problem, as you see it?

   _____

   _____

4. Exactly what are you asking Dr. Blau to do?

   _____

   _____

5. How soon does this problem need to be solved?

   _____

   _____

6. The solution to this problem should be _____

   _____

   _____

OBSERVER #1, #2, and #3

1. What are the main issue(s) for Dr. McVoy?

    _____

    _____

2. What are the main issue(s) for Dr. Lagos?

    _____

    _____

3. Exactly what is the problem, as you see it?

    _____

    _____

4. Exactly what is Dr. Blau being asked to do?

    _____

    _____

5. How soon does this problem need to be solved?

    _____

6. Is Dr. Blau the one to solve it?   _____

    If not, who is?_____

7. The solution to this problem should be _____

    _____

Step 2. Taking Action (20 minutes)

In this step, Drs. Blau, McVoy, and Lagos will each role-play their parts while the observers take notes. The observers will be giving feedback later.

Drs. Blau, McVoy, and Lagos should assume that the problem has been sufficiently aired and that they are now ready to move into some type of problem-resolution stage. Accordingly, Dr. Blau should direct his efforts (and hopefully their efforts, too) toward a solution to this problem. Drs. McVoy and Lagos are still somewhat upset about the issue and with each other, though they would probably rationally agree that a solution should be the major outcome of their meeting. At the end of the role play, if no solution has been reached, Dr. Blau should resolve the problem and tell Drs. McVoy and Lagos about his decision.

The observers will use the following page on which to take their notes.

OBSERVER'S NOTES

1. If you had to characterize Dr. McVoy in this session, would you characterize her as (choose one of the following):

   _____ hostile   _____ withdrawn

   _____ defensive   _____ evasive

   _____ ready to cooperate   _____ other _____

2. If you had to characterize Dr. Lagos in this session, would you characterize him as (choose one of the following):

   _____ hostile   _____ withdrawn

   _____ defensive   _____ evasive

   _____ ready to cooperate   _____ other _____

3. Does Dr. Blau ever define the problem, or try to get Drs. McVoy and Lagos to agree on exactly what the problem is?

   _____

   _____

   _____

4. Does Dr. Blau seem to have a plan in mind, or to be using a system, to mediate this conflict?

   _____

   _____

   If so, what is it? _____

   _____

(Continued on next page)

5. What specific techniques (words, body language, threats, praise, etc.) is Dr. Blau using with Dr. McVoy to attempt to settle this problem?

_____

_____

_____

6. Whom does Dr. Blau feel should solve the problem?

_____

_____

_____

Step 3. Debriefing (20 minutes)

Within your small group discuss the role play you have just completed. Discuss the role play by contrasting your approach to problem solving with the one listed below. Observers should also give feedback on which actions of Dr. Blau were helpful in solving the conflict and which actions were not helpful. As the purpose of this simulation is to acquaint participants with managing an institutional community, most of the comments should focus on Dr. Blau.

After reading this problem situation, an experienced administrator suggested that Dr. Blau should have taken the following steps:

1. Overcome or change Drs. McVoy's and/or Lagos's attitude(s) into ones of willingness to cooperate;

2. Come to some type of agreement on the definition of the problem;

3. Determine from Lagos and McVoy their perception of who should solve the problem;

4. Refer the problem to the lowest level possible for solution (i.e., Drs. Lagos and McVoy, or Dr. O'Sullivan); and

5. Set a time limit for the solution of the problem and report back to you.

This suggested "solution" is based on the following principles:

1. An attitude of willingness to cooperate is more helpful than one of defensiveness, hostility, etc.;

2. An exact definition of the problem is a necessary antecedent to the solution of the problem;

3. Solving a problem at the lowest level possible in the organization will help to insure the acceptance of the solution;

4. Delegation can be just as important as mediation.

FRAME IV

DELEGATING WORK TO SUBORDINATES

You finally were able to get away for some lunch and a fairly restful, quiet hour by yourself. You return to your office and see on your desk a basket marked "To Be Delegated." You pull out the papers in that basket and realize that these are fairly urgent matters which should probably be delegated to your subordinates. Some of them are addressed to you, and some are left over from the former superintendent. You know that you need to delegate each problem to one person and provide adequate instructions. You smile to yourself as you remember one of your professors saying for the 500th time, "Beware of the administrator who directs but does not delegate or who delegates but does not direct."

Step 1. Collective Executive (20 minutes)

In this step, each of you will play Dr. Blau. Read each of the following items and decide if it should be delegated to someone. If it should be delegated, refer to the organizational charts in the Introduction to determine who should receive it. Also include a note explaining what should be done and a deadline. Write on the bottom of each item.

When everyone has completed this step, proceed to the next step.

In-Basket #1

MEMORANDUM

TO: Dr. Tom Blau, Superintendent

FROM: Jim Lewis, Alcoholism Program Supervisor

RE: Program Update

DATE: July 9, 1978

Recently there has been a great deal of published research regarding a new treatment method for addicts that are institutionalized. The first time I came across the material I realized that this was the kind of thing we needed to do at Thronateeska. I have been in contact with the Education Supervisor and she agrees that this is the direction that we need to be moving in. She has also agreed to support my efforts and actively participate in the program design.

I would appreciate a meeting with you at your earliest convenience in order to solidify the conceptual model.

ACTION TO BE TAKEN -- By whom? Deadline?

_____

_____

_____

_____

_____

_____

In-Basket #2

MEMORANDUM

TO: Robert Lagos, Clinical Director

FROM: Mary Hadi, Assistant Superintendent Administration

RE: Renovation of W-2 Unit

DATE: July 2, 1978

In reference to your question regarding the priority and status of the proposed renovation for W-2 Unit, I have been advised by General Services that supplies have been ordered and that construction should begin within the next two weeks.

As you realize, patients who are presently housed in the W-2 Unit will have to be transferred prior to any construction. I hope you also realize that patients cannot be made eligible for Medicaid reimbursement payments if they are housed in W-1 Unit. This unit is not Medicaid approved.

If there are any questions, please feel free to call me.

cc: Superintendent ✔
     Assistant Superintendent
     Medical General Services

ACTION TO BE TAKEN -- By whom? Deadline?

_____

_____

_____

_____

_____

In-Basket #3

MEMORANDUM

TO: Dr. Tom Blau, Superintendent

FROM: Tom Atkins, Psychiatric Aide

RE: Forensic Duty

DATE: July 9, 1978

    I feel that there is an injustice that needs to be corrected immediately. Over the past two months when I arrive for my regular shift (11 p.m. - 7 a.m.) and report to the Supervising Nurse, I am instructed to report to the Forensic Unit to talk to patients that have caused disturbances during the day. At first I did not mind this but it has caused me to neglect my regular patients for whom I care a great deal. I was not hired for Forensic duty. I would not have taken a job at Thronateeska if I had known that I would be working with criminal patients. It is dangerous and I have two stitches over my eye to prove it. It is wrong to hire someone for one job and then use them for another.

    I sincerely hope that you will take some immediate action on this matter.

ACTION TO BE TAKEN -- By whom? Deadline?

_____

_____

_____

_____

_____

_____

In-Basket #4

MEMORANDUM

TO: Dr. Tom Blau

FROM: Bud Dudley, Psychiatric Social Worker in
         Alcohol Program

RE: Social Work Training Grant

DATE: July 9, 1978

I have just been informed through an old contact in the University System that NIMH has money to fund the training for psychiatric social workers in experimental programs in institutional settings. Intent to apply for these funds must be made by August 15, 1978.

As you must be aware, our manpower requirements are critical in the Social Services Department. This kind of funding would allow us to beef up our staffing needs and accomplish many of the things we are so far behind on.

Please advise me directly if you would like for me to follow up on this funding.

ACTION TO BE TAKEN -- By whom? Deadline?

_____

_____

_____

_____

_____

In-Basket #5

Thronateeska State Hospital

To Whom It May Concern

Regarding Pt. Johnny Newhouse
Pt. 125-78-2485

Recently, I visited my brother the above named and was informed that I owed the hospital $1,842.00 for maintenance costs. I don't have no money like that and I was never given no idea from the first that I needed to pay for his keep. My welfare worker Mrs. Shanks in Bristol said maybe it was a good idea to write the hospital and explain my situation. My brother is a voluntary patient and has been very sick. I can see he is doing better though. Anyway before he got sick he and his wife left each other. She took everything he owned and moved to Iowa. He don't have nothing left. I am a widow with 4 children and can hardly make it on social security and welfare. I was made his guardian because there was no one else left.

Please do something for my brother. I love him and I want him well again.

May the good Lord Bless You

Margaret Hess
Margaret Hess

ACTION TO BE TAKEN -- By whom?   Deadline?

_____

_____

_____

_____

_____

In-Basket #6

MEMORANDUM

TO: Superintendent

FROM: Mary Hadi

RE: Installation of Cable T.V.

DATE: June 14, 1976

     All the bids for cable T.V. in all wards in the hospital have been received. The low bid was made by Florida T.V. Antenna Inc. Their bid is reasonable and money is available to cover the installation costs. All that is necessary to begin at this time is your decision to go ahead. Bids will not be binding after July 30, so I urge you to move now if you intend to. I am told by the engineers involved that costs will double after August 1, due to a new F.C.C. requirement. Please advise.

ACTION TO BE TAKEN -- By whom? Deadline?

_____

_____

_____

_____

_____

_____

In-Basket #7

TO   Superintendent Office

DATE   July 5, 1978   TIME   11:00 a.m.

WHILE YOU WERE OUT

M   Enfield

OF   Sewing Room

PHONE   904-633-3280

Area Code   Number   Extension

TELEPHONED	X	PLEASE CALL	
CALLED TO SEE YOU		WILL CALL AGAIN	
WANTS TO SEE YOU		URGENT	
	RETURNED YOUR CALL		

MESSAGE   Wants to know when it will

be appropriate to put curtains in

visitors room.

                           T.A.

                        OPERATOR

ACTION TO BE TAKEN -- By whom?   Deadline?

Step 2. Classifying Responses (15 minutes)

Now that you have written a response to each in-basket item, it is time to classify these items. Two useful ways of classifying administrative matters are:

--Do today/hold for tomorrow;

--Program/nonprogram.

The first obviously refers to setting priorities on myriad problems that come before an administrator. The second refers to those matters which affect or relate directly to patients (program) and to those which are ancillary to treatment of patients, such as maintenance of the grounds, personnel, etc. (nonprogram).

Look again at the recommended actions you developed for the in-basket items in this frame and classify them in each of these two classifications. That is, place the item number in one of the boxes below. Work by yourself. When all participants have finished this step, proceed to the next step.

	DO TODAY	HOLD FOR TOMORROW
PROGRAM		
NONPROGRAM		

Step 3. Comparing Responses (20 minutes)

Divide into groups of three or four. Work through the in-baskets, item by item, and compare your responses of Step 1 and classifications of Step 2 to each other's. Be sure to listen to each person's rationale for his/her decision.

Step 4. Debriefing (20 minutes)

The debriefing will take a different format from earlier debriefings. After you reached some consensus in the prior step, compare your responses with those listed below.

How did you do?

_____

Do you disagree with some of the responses?

_____

If so, which ones?

_____

Actually all the in-basket items in this frame should not have come to the superintendent's attention or at least should require no response from him.

1. The memo from Jim Lewis, alcohol program supervisor, is inappropriate because it violates the regular chain of command. It should be returned to the assistant superintendent medical, with a note to Mr. Lewis thanking him and saying this memo had been rerouted to the assistant superintendent medical and that you're looking forward to meeting him.

   HOLD FOR TOMORROW - PROGRAM

2. The memo from Mary Hadi is for information purposes only and is not asking for a decision by the superintendent. But it might be helpful to you, the superintendent, to know what the plans for W-1 are currently.

   HOLD FOR TOMORROW - NONPROGRAM

3. Tom Atkins's kind of communication is appropriate between line and top staff echelons. However, the means in this case is inappropriate. A memo should not be used. Either a personal letter (better) or confidential memo (worse) is appropriate and satisfies the purpose. Action on this information should be a personal investigation by the superintendent. Mr. Atkins should receive a memo from you which tells Mr. Atkins his memo has been received and that the policy is to be reviewed.

   TODAY - NONPROGRAM

4. Not only is Dudley's memo inappropriate because it violates the chain of command, but it does not bear the initials of the sender. It should be returned to the alcohol program supervisor.

   HOLD FOR TOMORROW - PROGRAM

5. This Newhouse letter should not have been given to the superintendent. A letter of this type should be routinely routed for response and action to the business manager.

   HOLD FOR TOMORROW - PROGRAM

6. This cable T.V. memo has been collecting dust for over two years. It requires no decision because all relevant dates have passed.

7. A telephone message like this should not be passed on to an administrator for a decision. It would be worth your while, however, to find out if Dr. Rogers insisted upon making decisions like these. Then you could make the determination if you wished to continue this practice or not.

   TODAY - NONPROGRAM

FRAME V

STAFF PROBLEM SOLVING

Your second day as superintendent of Thronateeska is almost over. You have had to switch gears many times during the day, to meet several new problems. Each problem, it seems, has called for a new skill on your part. While you were working with your last set of memos, your administrative assistant put two more memoranda on your desk. You read these memos.

MEMORANDUM

TO: Dr. Tom Blau, Superintendent

FROM: David Webster, Director of the *DW*
        Division of Mental Health

RE: Misallocation of Funds

DATE: July 8, 1978

Prior to your arrival we had talked about a very serious budget situation at Thronateeska. At that time I did not get all the details, but apparently it had something to do with the misutilization of $175,000. I do not need to remind you that this is an election year. Elections are only 4 months away, and this kind of situation could have the most severe political consequences.

Please advise me on this situation as soon as possible. I trust it will be remedied immediately.

MEMORANDUM

TO: Tom Blau, Superintendent

FROM: Mark Hinson, Division of
        Social Services Department

RE: Departmental Funding

DATE: July 9, 1978

I have just been astounded to find out that money appropriated to my department was misdirected and misutilized by the business manager. It is difficult to believe that $175,000 generated by my department as reimbursement money for services as required by Social Security could be touched without my knowledge, much less be utilized for paving a street on the hospital grounds through the doctor's quarters. I do not believe that the error was intentional but I do believe it indicates a serious problem.

The consequences of this error will result in an audit exception which will be embarrassing to the hospital all the way to the governor. It also jeopardizes federal funding for next fiscal year. It also keeps the Social Service Department from fulfilling a large portion of legislative mandate.

cc: Assistant Superintendent, Medical
     Assistant Superintendent, Administration

A quick phone call to the assistant superintendent of administration confirms the error. According to the business manager, the error resulted from a weak battery in his pocket calculator, which he didn't notice as he was up very late the night he was working on the budget. The $175,000 was shown as surplus money which could be utilized for hospital improvements.

Step 1. Assigning Roles and Conducting the Meeting (30 minutes)

The instructor will assign roles to individuals. Each of you will participate in a staff meeting in which you will attempt to develop a way to solve the problems of the misallocated $175,000. Read the role description on the following pages for the role that has been assigned to you. When all participants have read their roles, begin the staff meeting by going around the circle and introducing yourself and stating how you feel about the subject under discussion. When each of you has introduced him/herself, then the superintendent should begin the meeting.

The roles are:

Superintendent - Dr. Tom Blau;

Assistant Superintendent, Administration - Mary Hadi;

Assistant Superintendent, Medical - Dr. Jack O'Sullivan;

Social Service Director - Mark Hinson;

Business Manager - Max Lawrence.

Role Description for <u>Dr. Tom Blau</u>, Superintendent

    Remember that this is only your second day on the job, so you
don't know the other members of the staff as well as you'd like to.
Also remember that the staff has had a long day, and they are probably
tired and thus will give in even more to the tendency to hide their
errors. You are very concerned about the $175,000 error, for you
understand its ramifications to the hospital--both internally and
externally (i.e., politically). You must balance this concern for the
hospital itself with your concern for the staff involved. Your job
during this staff meeting is to allow everyone to air his/her views on
what should be done and then decide what is the best way to handle the
situation. Remember that the ultimate decision is yours--and you, and
the entire staff, must live with the consequences of your decision.

Role Description for <u>Mary Hadi</u>, Assistant Superintendent,
    Administration

    You would like to fire the business manager, as you see him as
being totally responsible for the error and incompetent in the duties
of the position he occupies. Yet you also know that he reports
directly to you, and so you are ultimately responsible for the $175,000
error. You also know that if you are forced to make up this $175,000
error by slashing other areas of the budget, those who have been cut
will be angry with you.
    In relation to the hospital's relationship with the state office
of the Division of Mental Health and the legislature, you feel that a
complete public disclosure should be made, both of the error itself and
of the steps that have been taken to insure that such an error does not
happen again. But such a disclosure must not implicate you in the
blame. You would much prefer that Max Lawrence take all the heat. You
really have no solution to propose, as you are caught between wanting
Max Lawrence to be punished and wanting to keep your reputation clean.

Role Description for <u>Dr. Jack O'Sullivan</u>, Assistant Superintendent, Medical

   You have been employed at the hospital for many years and know Max Lawrence well. You and he often play golf together, and you do not want to see your friend get hurt. You have heard talk of a full disclosure, but you want a full coverup of the incident. You are afraid that such a disclosure may lead to investigations which may ultimately involve all the hospital. While you know of no wrongdoing in the hospital as a whole, you think that such an investigation could be disruptive to the standard operating procedures and possibly the morale of the hospital as a whole. Accordingly, you advocate a full coverup.

Role Description for <u>Mark Hinson</u>, Director of the Social Services Department

   You have been at the hospital only a few years. You are tired of the medical doctors having all the say in the operation of the hospital. You think that Max Lawrence is in total sympathy with the doctors regarding the preservation of the status quo. You know you would not have been included in this meeting if you had not written the memorandum to Dr. Blau. This is precisely the reason why you wrote it.

   When you first came to the hospital, you also made an error in computing your budget request. Had this error not been caught, your department could have had its funds slashed in half. But the error was caught, and you attributed it to youthfulness on your part. You would never make such an error again. If mention of your error is made, you intend to threaten to go to the press. This meeting is to discuss Max Lawrence, not you! You advocate at the very least a full public disclosure, and you'd be delighted if Dr. Blau would go so far as to fire Mr. Lawrence.

Role Description for <u>Max Lawrence</u>, Business Manager

    You have been employed at Thronateeska for 18 years and have
received several letters of commendation from past administrators. You
are concerned about the security of your job and the loss of your
retirement benefits. You have a short time left until retirement, and
you would like to retire rather than be fired.

    Dr. O'Sullivan has been your friend for many years. You often
play golf together. You know that he will come to your aid in this
meeting, and you are counting on him to protect you from attack by the
other members of the staff. You know that Mary Hadi is very mad at
you--and you also know that, as her direct subordinate, she can be held
as responsible as you for the $175,000 mistake.

    Mark Hinson, you have heard, wrote a memorandum to Dr. Blau about
the error. This is why he is sitting in on this meeting, you suspect,
although you are not sure and do not want to take any chances. You
recall that when Mark first came on board, he made a silly error in
computing his department's budget request for the upcoming year. Had
one of your staff not caught that error, Mark's department could have
lost up to half its funds.

    What is uppermost in your mind during this meeting is your job.
You are willing to accept an official reprimand, although you feel the
mistake was really due to the mechanical error of machines and not your
own error. Above all, you do not want to lose your job!

Step 2. Debriefing (20 minutes)

Staying within your same group, but dropping your roles, answer the following questions:

1. What was the decision reached by Dr. Blau? Do you agree with his decision? If not, what would you suggest?

2. How did Dr. Blau communicate his decision to the staff? Do you agree with his method of communication? If not, how would you have done it?

3. Is it better to castigate a good employee? Or is it better to openly admit mistakes and go on from there?

4. Below is one experienced mental health administrator's reaction to this situation. Read it, compare it to how your group handled the situation, and discuss the differences and similarities.

Secrecy with regard to mistakes is generally unwise; coverup is even worse. Anyone can make mistakes. It serves no real purpose to reprimand or castigate an excellent employee for a legitimate mistake. On the contrary, in fact, it often is more embarrassing and may possibly take away his initiative. Just the fact that he knows that you know will make him more careful in the future.

Admit mistakes openly and encourage your associates and employees to do likewise. Set the example and gain the respect of your employees and minimize the opportunities of the saboteurs. Open information sharing can clear communication channels and lead to the creation of a healthy organizational environment.

If you were a gutsy administrator in this situation, you would document your actions very carefully and forward a copy of these actions to the state office.

RELATED READINGS

Belknap, I. Human problems of a state mental hospital. New York: Basic Books, 1956.

Blau, P. M. Bureaucracy in modern society. New York: Random House, 1966.

Caudill, W. A. The psychiatric hospital as a small society. Cambridge, Mass.: Harvard University Press, 1958.

Ennis, B., & Siegel, L. The rights of mental patients. New York: Avon Books, 1973.

Fisher, W. Human services: The third revolution in mental health. Port Washington, N. Y.: Alfred Publishing Co., 1974.

Goffman, E. Asylums: Essays on the social situation of mental patients and other inmates. Chicago: Aldine Publishing Co., 1962.

Greenblatt, M., Sharaf, M. R., & Stone, E. M. Dynamics of institutional change: The hospital in transition. Pittsburgh: University of Pittsburgh Press, 1971.

Greenblatt, M., Levinson, D. J., & Williams, R. (Eds.). The patient and the mental hospital. New York: Glencoe, 1957.

Smith, C. G., & King, J. A. Mental hospitals: A study in organizational effectiveness. Lexington, Mass.: Lexington Books, 1975.

Stanton, A., & Schwarz, M. The mental hospital. New York: Basic Books, 1954.